READER'S DIGEST

FIRST AID

READER'S
DIGEST

FIRST AID

First aid consultant
Sheena Meredith MB BS MRCS (ENG) LRCP (LOND)

Published by **The Reader's Digest Association Limited**
London • New York • Sydney • Montreal

Emergency procedures

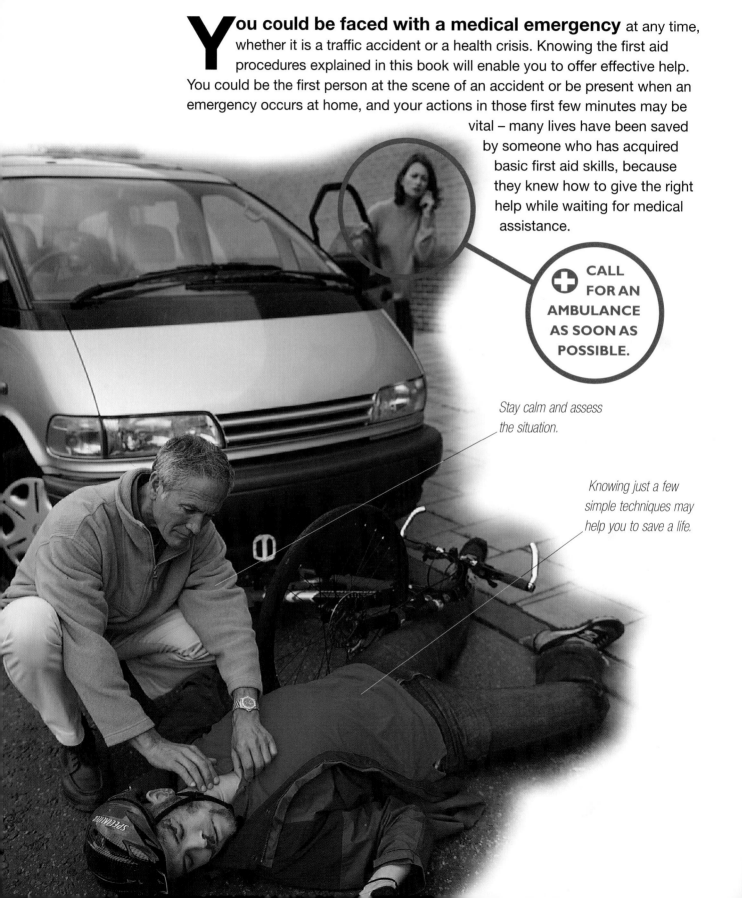

You could be faced with a medical emergency at any time, whether it is a traffic accident or a health crisis. Knowing the first aid procedures explained in this book will enable you to offer effective help. You could be the first person at the scene of an accident or be present when an emergency occurs at home, and your actions in those first few minutes may be vital – many lives have been saved by someone who has acquired basic first aid skills, because they knew how to give the right help while waiting for medical assistance.

➕ **CALL FOR AN AMBULANCE AS SOON AS POSSIBLE.**

Stay calm and assess the situation.

Knowing just a few simple techniques may help you to save a life.

If you keep calm and follow some basic first aid principles you can greatly improve the condition of almost any victim in an accident or crisis.

In any emergency situation there is much that can be done safely by the untrained or inexperienced bystander, but the first thing is always to get help quickly – wherever possible ask someone else to call the emergency services, and to come back to confirm that he or she has done so.

Keep a well-stocked first aid kit at home and in the car.

Pause for a moment to assess the situation. Make sure that you are not putting yourself in danger – you will be no help to the victim if you become a casualty, too. For example, if you are at the scene of a road accident and in a separate vehicle, switch on your hazard warning lights to warn other vehicles and, if possible, ask someone to warn approaching traffic.

Once the scene is safe, you can assess the victim – if there are multiple victims, you will need to decide who is the most seriously injured and treat those with life-threatening conditions first. If the victim is unconscious, follow the ABC procedure (see page 7).

If the victim is not breathing, he or she must be resuscitated immediately in order to maintain heartbeat and breathing (see pages 10–11), and action may be required in order to stem major bleeding (see pages 32–33 and 34–35).

There are many emergencies that occur at home, at work or during the course of daily life. Recognizing the signs of major medical emergencies such as a heart attack, stroke or diabetic coma, and knowing what to do until medical attention is available could save someone's life.

In many other circumstances, the victim may be in pain, confused or distressed. You can use basic first aid skills to relieve the injury and make the person more comfortable.

Whatever the circumstance, it is important to remain calm and reassuring. Familiarity with the basic first aid procedures will make this easier – and knowing what not to do will ensure that your first aid assistance is safe.

Priorities in an emergency:

- Call or send for help.
- Stop to assess the situation before taking action.
- Make sure it is safe to approach the scene.
- Ensure that victims and any bystanders are protected from immediate danger.
- In traffic accidents, turn off the ignition and check the handbrake of all vehicles involved.
- Be alert to potential dangers such as smoke and gas or petrol leakage.
- Assess the victims and treat life-threatening injuries first.

Basic life support chart

The victim has collapsed

Check response to a gentle shake and loud command

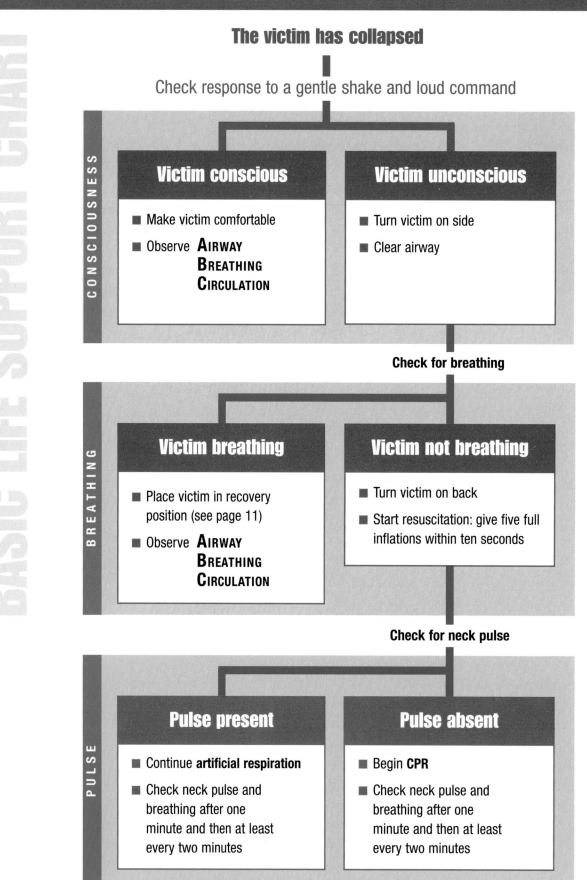

CONSCIOUSNESS

Victim conscious

- Make victim comfortable
- Observe **A**IRWAY **B**REATHING **C**IRCULATION

Victim unconscious

- Turn victim on side
- Clear airway

Check for breathing

BREATHING

Victim breathing

- Place victim in recovery position (see page 11)
- Observe **A**IRWAY **B**REATHING **C**IRCULATION

Victim not breathing

- Turn victim on back
- Start resuscitation: give five full inflations within ten seconds

Check for neck pulse

PULSE

Pulse present

- Continue **artificial respiration**
- Check neck pulse and breathing after one minute and then at least every two minutes

Pulse absent

- Begin **CPR**
- Check neck pulse and breathing after one minute and then at least every two minutes

ABC

Emergency procedures

In a life-threatening emergency, the strict priorities are to:

- Make the area safe if necessary

- Observe the ABC of first aid according to the basic life-support chart (see left)

- Treat for severe bleeding (see page 34)

AIRWAY

The recovery position is the only safe position for an unconscious person. Lie the person on one side, with the head and neck tilted back to keep the airway clear. Check and remove any obstruction (see page 8).
RECOVERY POSITION, SEE PAGE 11

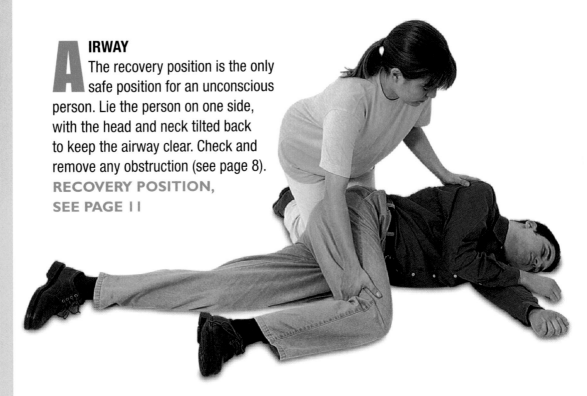

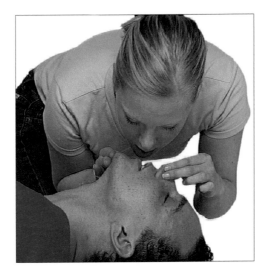

BREATHING

If the victim is not breathing, artificial respiration is given mouth to mouth to ventilate the lungs and provide vital oxygen to the tissues.
RESUSCITATION, SEE PAGE 10

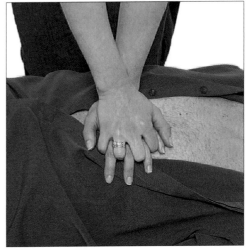

CIRCULATION

If the victim's heart is not beating, there will be no circulation of blood and he or she will die unless CPR, cardiopulmonary resuscitation, is given.
CPR, SEE PAGE 13

Airway, breathing and pulse

AIRWAY CHECK

In an emergency first check for any obstruction of the airway and then position the person to keep the airway open. When a person is unconscious, he or she cannot cough or swallow. Any food, fluid, vomit or blood can cause a fatal blockage of the airway which leads from the mouth and nose to the lungs.

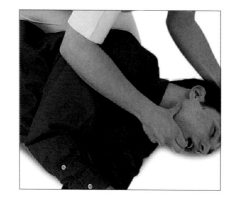

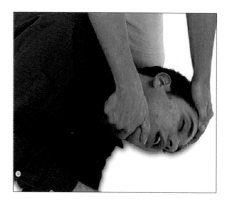

1 Look inside the mouth and if necessary use two fingers to check inside for anything that could block the airway. Remove any obvious obstructions but DO NOT try to probe the back of the throat. Leave any dentures in place unless they are broken.

2 Gently tilt back the head and bring the chin forwards by supporting the jaw. This will keep the airway open and prevent the tongue from blocking it. Ensure that the face is inclined slightly downwards to aid the drainage of any fluids.

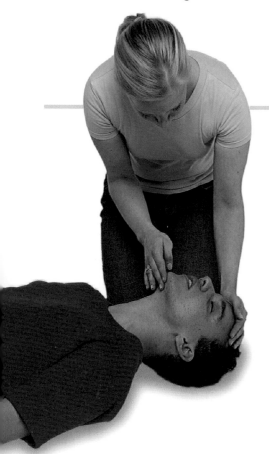

BREATHING CHECK

Look for rising movements of the chest or abdomen, listen for breathing sounds and feel for air coming from the victim's mouth or nose on your cheek. Keep looking, listening and feeling for up to ten seconds and be alert for very shallow breathing. If breathing is absent, give five quick breaths of artificial respiration (see page 10) and follow with a pulse check (see opposite).

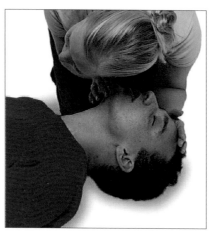

2 Lean down with your face close to the casualty's mouth. Look along the chest for movement whilst listening for sounds of breathing and feeling for the movement of breath against your cheek.

1 Check breathing while holding the airway open (see page 7).

PULSE CHECK

The pulse is a pressure wave in the arteries created by the beating of the heart. It can be used to check the state of the circulation: if there is no pulse, the heart has stopped and the victim needs immediate cardiopulmonary resuscitation (see page 13). It does not matter where on the body you take a pulse, but the carotid artery in the neck is usually easier to find when a victim is unconscious. If a victim is breathing and conscious the radial pulse, on the inside of the wrist, is the better place to check. A healthy adult pulse rate is between 60 to 80 beats per minute. It is naturally faster in children.

✚ **IF BREATHING OR PULSE ARE ABSENT, CALL AN AMBULANCE IMMEDIATELY.**

For an adult or child
The pulse is checked over the carotid artery, which can be felt on the neck, on either side of the windpipe. Feel for the pulse for up to ten seconds. If the pulse is absent, there is no need to check for breathing because the victim cannot breathe when the heart has stopped beating – begin CPR (see page 13) at once.

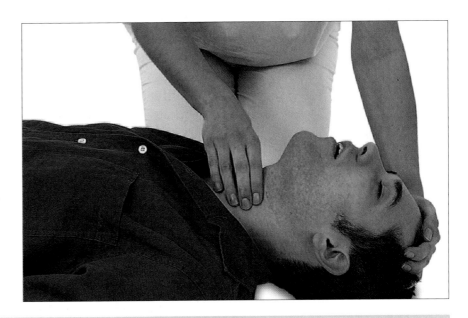

For a baby
If the pulse in the neck is hard to find, use the pulse in the inside of the upper arm. With your first and middle fingers feel for the pulse in the groove between the two upper arm muscles.

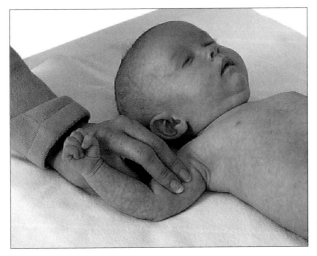

Resuscitation

Breathing and pulse checks

- Breathing and pulse checks should be made every two minutes during resuscitation to see whether the victim is recovering

- The breathing and pulse rates of any unconscious victim should be checked frequently for any changes in his or her condition

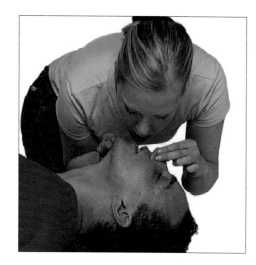

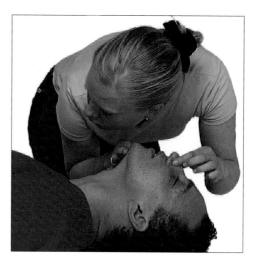

1 Kneel beside the victim and tilt the head back gently to keep the airway open (see page 8). Place two fingers under the chin to support the jaw in this position. Pinch the victim's nose with your thumb and first finger. Take a deep breath and seal your lips around the victim's mouth. Blow into the victim's airway for about two seconds – watch for the chest to rise.

2 Draw back for about four seconds turning your head to the side to watch the chest falling. Give a repeat inflation and then check the pulse (see page 9). If you find a pulse, continue to breathe for the victim, checking the pulse after every ten breaths. If there is no pulse, start CPR (cardiopulmonary resuscitation, see page 13).

For a baby or child

Use the same pattern of inflations for a child as for an adult, but use shorter breaths and pause as soon as the chest rises.
For a baby or infant, seal your lips around the mouth and the nose before inflating the chest, and stop breathing out as soon as the baby's chest rises.

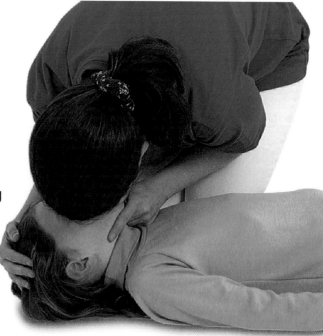

Recovery position

The recovery position is a safe position in which to place an unconscious casualty. It protects from injury by stopping the victim from rolling over, and ensures that the airway stays open and fluids – blood, saliva or vomit – can drain away without risk of choking.

➕ **CALL AN AMBULANCE IMMEDIATELY.**

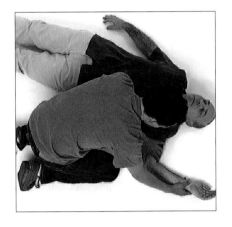 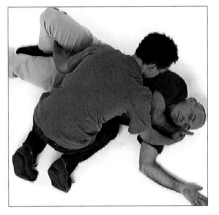 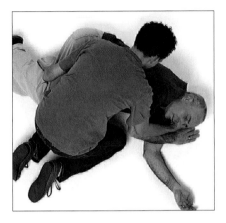

1 Kneel at the side of the victim, straighten the legs and place the arm nearest to you at a right angle to the body, with the forearm at a right angle to the upper arm.

2 Place the victim's other arm across the chest and support the cheek on the back of the hand. Bend the opposite knee upwards and pull to roll the victim towards you.

3 Support and protect the victim's head while rolling over. Keep the knee bent to prevent the victim from rolling too far.

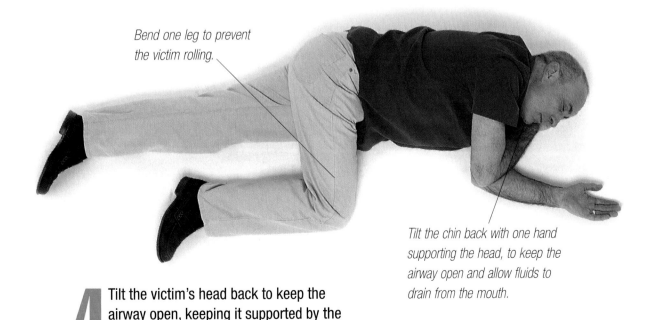

Bend one leg to prevent the victim rolling.

Tilt the chin back with one hand supporting the head, to keep the airway open and allow fluids to drain from the mouth.

4 Tilt the victim's head back to keep the airway open, keeping it supported by the back of the victim's hand. Check pulse and breathing regularly until medical help arrives.

Cardiac compression

Action to take if someone's heart stops

If no pulse is present, and therefore there is no circulation of blood around the body, the tissues are likely to die of oxygen starvation within three to four minutes.

- External cardiac compression should begin along with mouth-to-mouth respiration (see page 10) as soon as the pulse is discovered to be absent. These two techniques together are known as CPR (cardiopulmonary resuscitation, see page 13)

- Chest compressions must always be combined with mouth-to-mouth respiration

- Compression is over the lower half of the breastbone

1 Kneel beside the victim and if necessary roll him or her onto the back. Find the lower end of the ribcage and run your first two fingers inwards until you find the bottom of the breastbone. Place your index finger at this point as a marker. Place the heel of your other hand on the breastbone just above this finger and maintain this position.

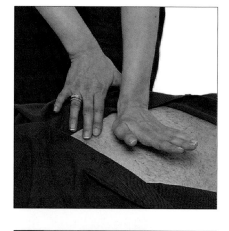

2 Move the other hand on top of the first and interlace your fingers. Lean forwards with your shoulders over the victim. Keeping your arms straight, push down, aiming to press the lower breastbone down by about one-third of the depth of the chest. Release the pressure without removing your hands. Repeat 15 times at a rate of 100 thrusts per minute (almost two per second), then give mouth-to-mouth respiration (see page 13).

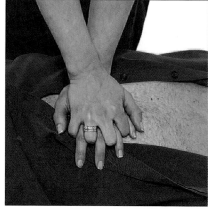

Grasp your lower hand with the fingers of your upper one.

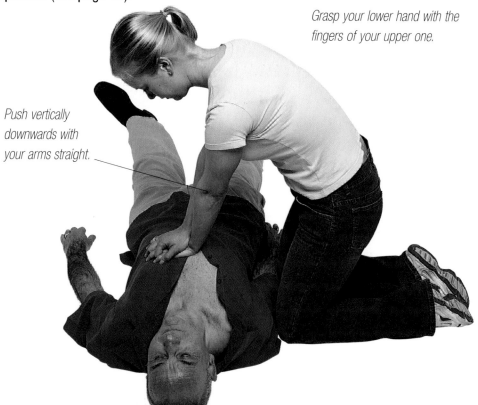

Push vertically downwards with your arms straight.

CPR Cardiopulmonary resuscitation

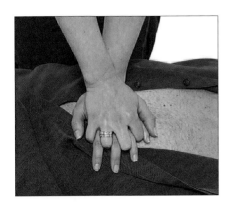

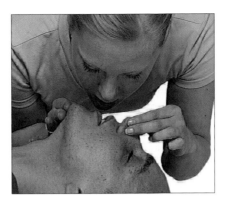

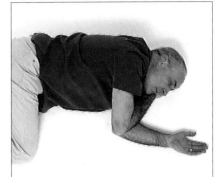

1 Following a steady series of 15 chest compressions (see page 12), give two breaths of mouth-to-mouth respiration (see page 10). Repeat this cycle, giving two breaths after each 15 chest compressions, until help arrives. If there are two rescuers, one can give the compressions and the other mouth-to-mouth respiration.

2 After one full minute of CPR, hold the victim's head in the open airway position (see page 8) and recheck for a neck pulse (see page 9). If the pulse is present, do not continue with compressions. Check breathing and if necessary carry on with respiration until normal breathing returns or medical help arrives.

3 If the victim regains a pulse and is breathing unassisted but remains unconscious, place him or her in the recovery position (see page 11). Check pulse and breathing regularly until help arrives, and be prepared to start CPR again if necessary.

CPR FOR BABIES AND CHILDREN

Use adult CPR techniques on children aged over eight years, unless they are particularly small for their age. For babies and children, you need to give gentler chest thrusts and very gentle breaths.

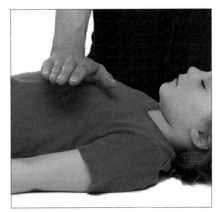

For a baby
Give breaths by sealing your lips around the baby's mouth and nose (see page 10). Place two fingers one finger's width below an imaginary line between the baby's nipples. Give chest compressions with the fingers only, at a rate of five compressions to one breath.

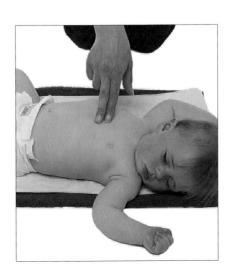

For a child (age 1–7)
Use one hand only to compress the chest and perform cycles of five chest compressions to one breath. Monitor pulse and breathing between each cycle, as for adults.

First aid kit

Every home and car should carry a well-stocked first aid kit which is checked regularly – supplies should be replenished when they are used or become out of date. Keep the kit in a clean, dry place where it is readily accessible when needed.

You can buy first aid kits from most pharmacists, or you can make up your own, provided that you keep it in a container with a well-fitting lid, that is both clean and watertight. A first aid kit should be clearly marked so that anyone can find it easily in an emergency.

Basic contents

- adhesive dressings (plasters)
- sterile dressings
- bandages in various sizes including triangular bandages
- dressing tape
- disposable latex gloves
- safety pins or bandage clips
- eye pads
- scissors
- antiseptic cream or spray
- cotton gauze swabs
- cotton wool for padding (not to be placed directly on a wound)
- notebook and pencil
- tweezers

bandages in various sizes

antiseptic spray for cleaning wounds

safety pins

cotton gauze swabs for cleaning and padding

notebook to record observations

adhesive tape to hold dressings in place

latex gloves for hygiene and protection

antiseptic cream

scissors for cutting bandages

antiseptic wipes to clean wounds and skin

adhesive dressings for small wounds

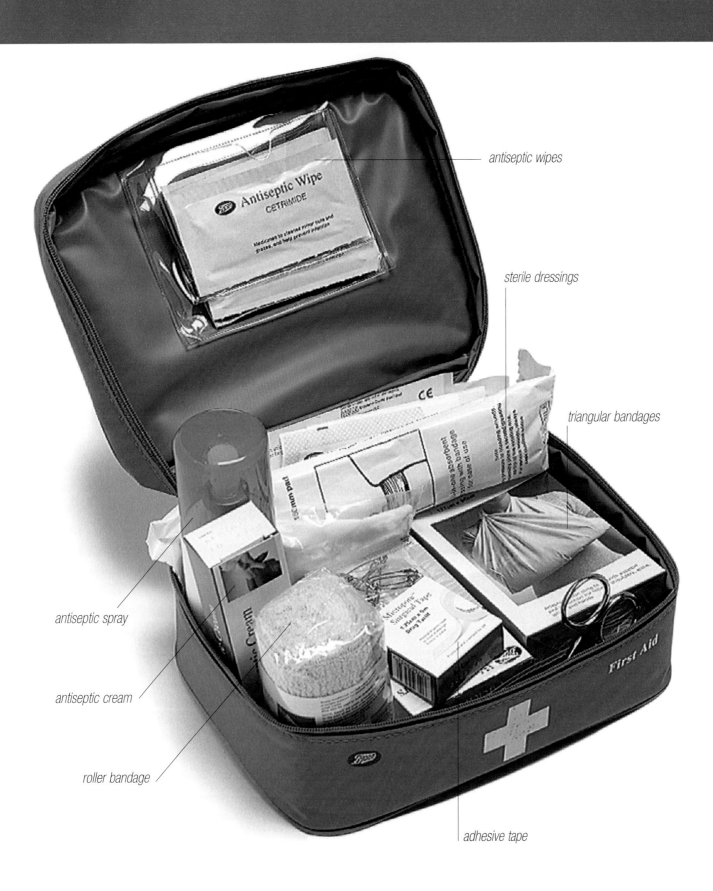

antiseptic wipes

sterile dressings

triangular bandages

antiseptic spray

antiseptic cream

roller bandage

adhesive tape

First Aid

Abdominal injury

Assessing the injury

- The abdominal cavity contains the stomach, liver, spleen, intestines, kidneys and some major blood vessels. Damage may occur without any obvious external wounds

- Careful assessment is needed to detect internal injuries which may lead to life-threatening collapse

What to look for:

- Pale, clammy skin
- Rapid, weak pulse
- Pain, confusion or collapse
- Bleeding from orifices, particularly the mouth

1 Help the victim to lie down in the most comfortable position possible. If a wound cuts across the abdomen, ease a cushion or rolled-up clothing under the knees to avoid straining the injury.

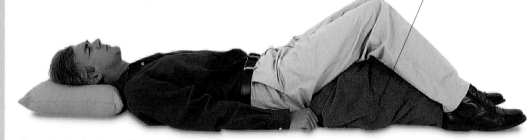

For wounds across the abdomen, place a soft support under the knees.

Do not raise the knees if the wound runs up and down the abdomen.

2 Loosen any tight clothing. If the wound is small, apply a sterile dressing fixed with a wide stretch-cotton bandage or wrap a towel around the abdomen.

Use a clean towel if there is no dressing to hand.

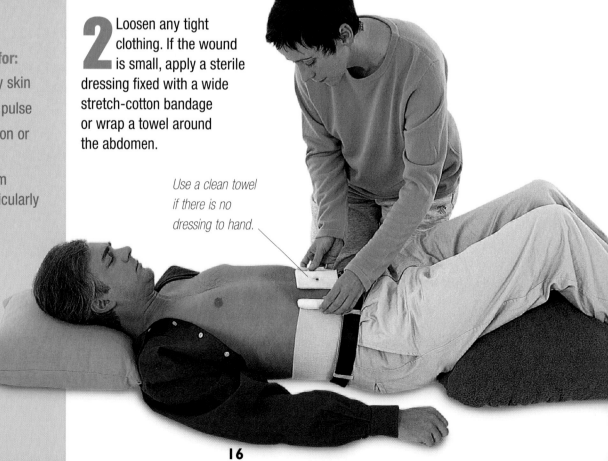

3 If internal organs are visible through the wound, do not touch or try to put them back in place. Cover the wound with plastic film or a plastic bag to prevent the intestine from drying out, or use a sterile, non-stick dressing moistened with a damp dressing or towel on top. If blood seeps through, cover with another dressing.

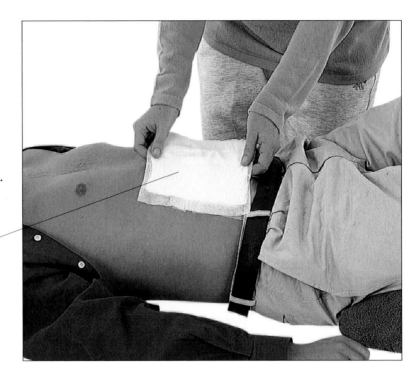

Use a damp dressing over the first dressing to keep it from drying out.

✚ **IF THE VICTIM COUGHS, SNEEZES OR VOMITS, APPLY LIGHT PRESSURE WITH YOUR PALMS ON TOP OF THE DRESSING TO PREVENT THE ABDOMINAL CONTENTS FROM PROTRUDING.**

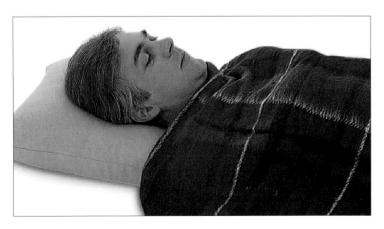

✚ **CALL AN AMBULANCE AS SOON AS POSSIBLE.**

4 Cover the victim lightly with a blanket or clothing to maintain the body temperature. If the victim is lying on a hot, cold or wet surface, ease a blanket, clothing or even newspapers under them. Take care to avoid any movement of the abdominal area.

5 While waiting for the ambulance, check the victim's airway, breathing and pulse every few minutes and monitor for signs of shock such as rapid and shallow breathing and weakening pulse (see page 85). Be prepared to give CPR (cardiopulmonary resuscitation, see page 13). If the wound is covered and secure, place an unconscious victim in the recovery position (see page 11).

Allergic reaction

Take action if any of the following occurs:

- Skin rash, blotchiness or redness
- Intense itching
- Abdominal pain, nausea or vomiting
- Breathing difficulty or wheezing
- Puffiness around the eyes
- Swelling, especially around the face

Almost anything can trigger an allergic reaction – common causes are food, drugs or medicines and insect stings. An allergic reaction can vary from an annoying but relatively harmless response, such as a skin rash, to severe and life-threatening collapse known as anaphylactic shock.

ANAPHYLACTIC SHOCK

Develops rapidly when allergic reaction causes swelling and constriction of the airway.
Signs include:

- Spreading skin reaction
- Swelling of the face
- Anxiety or panic
- Difficulty in breathing
- Rapid pulse

1 Help the victim to sit up in the most comfortable position to aid breathing.

2 Ask about previous allergic reactions. If the victim is aware of a severe allergy and carries emergency adrenaline (an Epi-Pen syringe), help the victim to use it.

3 If the the victim becomes unconscious, open the airway and check pulse and breathing (see pages 8–9). If necessary, be prepared to start resuscitation (see page 10). Place the victim in the recovery position (see page 11).

✚ **CALL AN AMBULANCE IMMEDIATELY**

Other reactions

Signs of less severe, localized allergic reactions include:

- Swelling of a body part (other than the face)
- Redness or heat under the skin
- Skin rash, itching or blistering
- Sneezing, runny eyes or nose

Offer first aid treatment for symptoms where possible. Advise the victim to seek medical advice if there is a history of allergic reaction or symptoms do not improve.

Ankle and foot injury

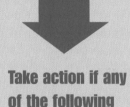

Take action if any of the following occurs:

- Pain in and around the injured area
- An open wound
- Inability to walk or to put weight on the foot
- Feeling faint or giddy
- Numbness in the foot or toes
- Loss of power and movement at the ankle joint

What to look for:

- Swelling around the joint

The most common ankle injury is caused by twisting the joint or from impact when jumping or falling from a height. The injury may be a sprain or a fracture (broken bone), but it can be difficult to decide the extent of the injury until an X-ray has been taken. To avoid the risk of further damage, treat all severe ankle injuries as possible fractures and advise the victim to seek medical advice as soon as possible.

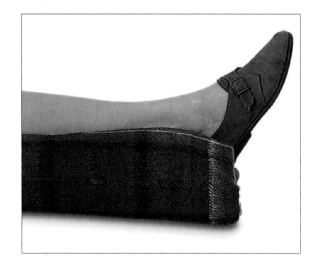

1 Help the victim to sit or lie down, avoiding moving or touching the injured joint. Carefully raise and support the injured leg in the most comfortable position for the victim.

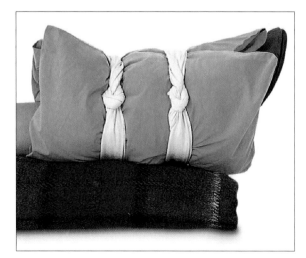

2 Carefully pad around the ankle using a soft pillow or light blanket held in place with two or three bandages. Reduce any swelling by applying an ice pack or cold compress (see page 31).

✚ **IF PAIN PERSISTS AND YOU SUSPECT A FRACTURE, TAKE THE VICTIM TO HOSPITAL. DO NOT GIVE ANY FOOD OR DRINK AS AN ANAESTHETIC MAY BE NEEDED.**

Arm and elbow injury

Take action if any of the following occurs:

- Pain in and around the injured area, often increased by movement
- Feeling cold and shivery
- Feeling faint and giddy
- Numbness in the extremities
- Loss of power and function in the joint

What to look for:
- Swelling

FOREARM

Arm injuries include dislocations of the elbow joint and fractures of one or more bones. An X-ray is often needed to confirm the diagnosis, and any serious injury should be treated as a possible fracture until medical advice has been obtained.

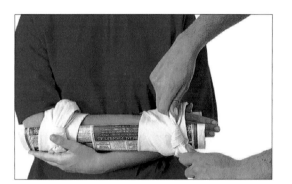

1 For a lower arm injury, gently support the arm and place a flattened, rolled newspaper under the forearm as a temporary splint. Secure it with a sling (see pages 28–29), keeping the fingers slightly higher than the elbow.

2 Check the pulse and colour of the fingertips every few minutes. If necessary, remove the bandages and splint and reposition them.
If the pulse cannot be felt, take the victim to hospital for urgent assessment.

ELBOW

Rest the injured arm on a soft support.

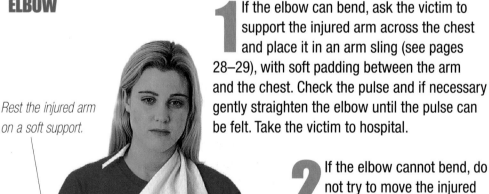

1 If the elbow can bend, ask the victim to support the injured arm across the chest and place it in an arm sling (see pages 28–29), with soft padding between the arm and the chest. Check the pulse and if necessary gently straighten the elbow until the pulse can be felt. Take the victim to hospital.

2 If the elbow cannot bend, do not try to move the injured limb. Ask the victim to lie down and place padding around the elbow to support it. Keep checking the pulse until the ambulance arrives.

✚ **CALL AN AMBULANCE. DO NOT BANDAGE THE ARM UNLESS THIS IS NECESSARY TO MOVE THE VICTIM TO SAFETY.**

Asthmatic attack

During an asthma attack, the airways are narrowed, restricting breathing. The muscles go into spasm, the mucous membrane lining swells, and thick, sticky mucus is produced. Attacks may be triggered by allergy, cold, exercise or infection, although often no trigger can be identified.

Take action if the following occurs:

- Difficulty in breathing, often, but not always, associated with wheezing or coughing

What to look for:

- Wheezing, especially when breathing out
- Coughing, especially at night
- Difficulty in talking
- Blue lips
- Anxiety

Asthma medication

Most asthmatics carry a 'reliever' inhaler so that they have access to treatment at the first sign of an attack. Inhalers usually have a blue cap and should ease symptoms within five to ten minutes. A plastic 'spacer' may be used to make it easier to breathe in the medicine

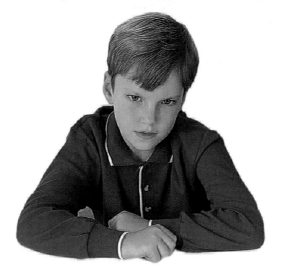

1 Help the victim into a comfortable position – sitting and leaning forwards on the arms often helps to reduce breathing effort. Ask the victim to breathe slowly and deeply, and offer frequent reassurance.

2 Help the victim to use a reliever inhaler if available, preferably through a 'spacer' device if the victim is a child. If the attack eases, another dose can be taken after five to ten minutes.

➕ **CALL AN AMBULANCE:**
- **IF THERE IS NO IMPROVEMENT AFTER 5–10 MINUTES.**
- **IF THE ATTACK IS GETTING WORSE DESPITE MEDICATION.**
- **IF THE VICTIM IS BECOMING EXHAUSTED.**
- **IF THE VICTIM COLLAPSES, STOPS BREATHING OR BECOMES UNCONSCIOUS.**

➕ **BE PREPARED TO START RESUSCITATION IF THE VICTIM STOPS BREATHING (SEE PAGE 10).**

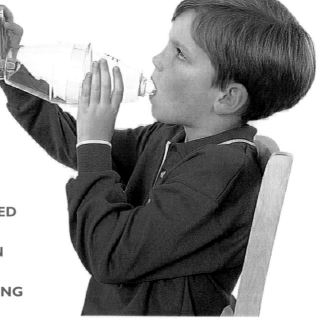

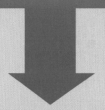

Back injury

Take action if the following occurs:

- Back pain, sometimes radiating down the outer leg

Call an ambulance if there is:

- Restricted movement in the lower limbs
- Loss of sensation or tingling or burning in the legs
- Headache
- Stiff neck
- Blurred or double vision
- Bloodstained urine (from internal bleeding)

What to look for:

- Any signs of recent injury
- Drowsiness or loss of consciousness

The back muscles can be injured by heavy lifting, a severe fall or by a sudden turn of the trunk area. The lower back is most commonly injured and the victim may also suffer painful muscle spasm. More rarely, the spine itself may be injured after a heavy fall or impact. If the pain is severe or accompanied by any of the symptoms listed on the left, seek urgent medical advice.

1 If the injury is obviously not serious, help the victim to rest in the most comfortable position, generally lying flat.

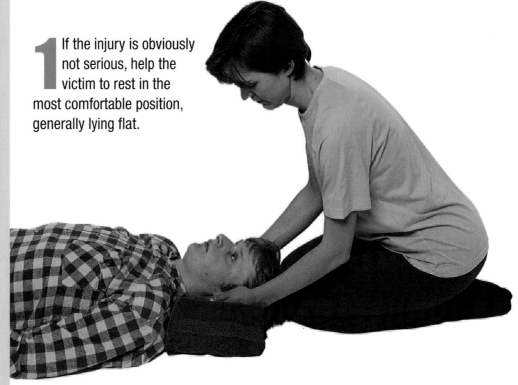

✚ **CALL AN AMBULANCE IMMEDIATELY IF THE INJURY IS ASSOCIATED WITH AN IMPACT OR SEVERE FALL, AND THE VICTIM IS CONSCIOUS. AVOID ANY MOVEMENT OF THE HEAD, NECK OR BACK.**

2 If there is soreness of the lower back after carrying a heavy load or after a sudden twisting movement, the victim should rest for up to an hour. This will help to ease the muscle spasm.

Bandages

Applying bandages and dressings is an important part of first aid. Sterile dressings come in various sizes and are made either with an absorbent surface for use on major wounds and to control bleeding, or with a non-adherent surface for use on burns or a weeping graze. Adhesive dressings are used for minor wounds and should be changed daily because the adhesive softens the skin and can delay healing. Roller bandages have many uses: to apply pressure, to control bleeding, support an injury and secure dressings on a wound.

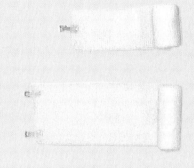

Adhesive dressings

Roller bandages

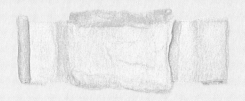

*Sterile wound dressings
and bandages*

Sterile combined dressing

Safety pins

Triangular bandage

*Sterile non-adherent
dry dressings*

*Adhesive
tape*

*Cotton gauze
swab*

Using a triangular bandage

- Use a triangular bandage to make a sling, or to tie a splint to a limb or to create a comfortable protective covering

- Secure dressings in place on a hand or foot wound with a triangular bandage. But remember that it will not supply enough pressure on its own to control any bleeding

- Use a triangular bandage for elbow and knee injuries. Support an injured elbow with the arm partly bent, if this is possible

HAND INJURY

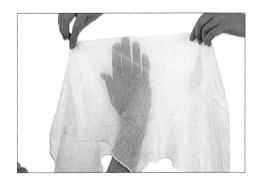

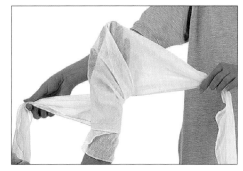

1 With the hand on an open triangular bandage – as above, or on a flat surface – bring the point over the injury.

2 Cross the ends around the wrist, covering the hand with the bandage. Make one full turn around the wrist.

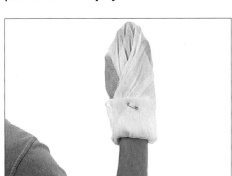

3 Tie the ends over the point, using a secure knot. Tuck the bandage ends around the wrist. Bring the point up over the knot and secure with a safety pin.

ELBOW INJURY

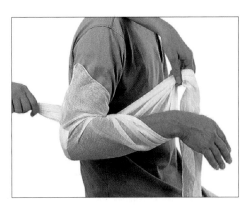

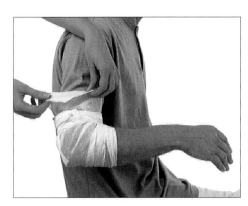

1 Place the bandage over the elbow with the point upwards and the base below the elbow on the outside of the lower arm.

2 Cross the ends behind the elbow, bring to the outside upper arm and tie with a secure knot. Bring the point down over the knot and pin.

KNEE INJURY

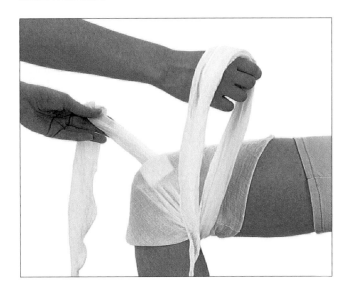

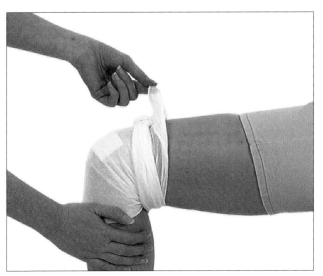

1 Cover the bent knee with the open triangular bandage, the point upwards and the base under the knee. Cross the ends behind the knee and up around the thigh.

2 Tie the ends above the knee in front, using a secure knot. Bring the point down over the knot and fasten it securely with a safety pin.

FOOT INJURY

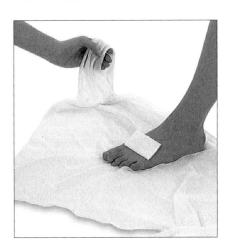

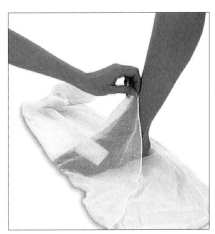

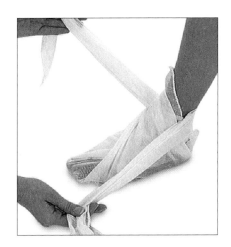

1 Place the foot on the open triangular bandage, with toes pointing towards the point.

2 Bring the point up as far as the ankle, covering the dressing and the whole foot.

3 Cross the ends around the ankle to secure the point. Tie a secure knot in the front. Bring the point down over the knot and pin to fix in position.

Bandaging head _triangular_

HEAD INJURY

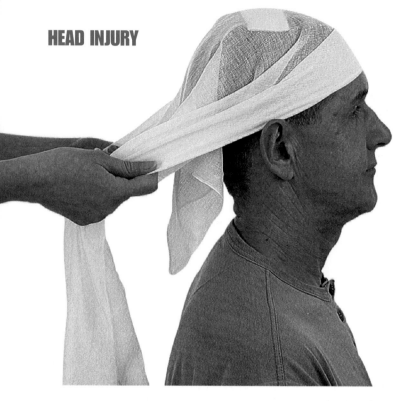

1 Fold a narrow hem inwards along the base to make a firm edge.

2 Place the hem around the forehead of the victim, with the point hanging down towards the back and the ends away from the head.

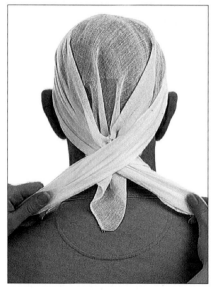

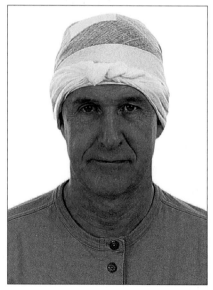

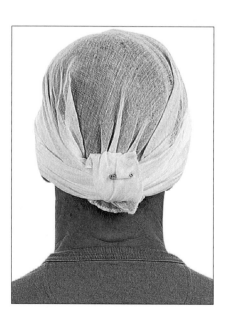

3 Carry the ends over the point, cross them, and return them around the head and back to the forehead.

4 Tie the ends with a secure knot, being careful not to tie too tightly and create excessive pressure.

5 Lift the point at the back of the head to cover the crossed ends, tuck it in and use a safety pin to secure.

Bandaging roller and tubular

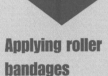

Applying roller bandages

- Position yourself facing the victim, on the injured side
- Place the bandage end against the skin, with the roll on top
- Unroll only a short length of bandage at a time
- Apply the bandage from the inner side of the body and work outwards
- Start the turns below the injury or wound, and work upwards
- When bandaging, cover two-thirds of each previous turn to hold the bandage firmly in place

SIMPLE SPIRAL BANDAGES FOR LIMBS

Roller bandages have four main uses: to support an injury, apply pressure, control bleeding, and secure a dressing. Widths vary from 2.5cm (1in) for fingers right up to 15cm (6in) for the trunk.

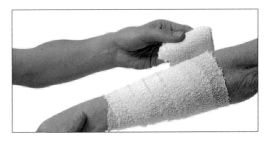

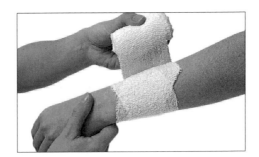

1 Start the bandage below the injury applying one or two turns in order to hold it in place.

2 Wind the bandage with a series of overlapping spiral turns around and up the limb.

3 Finish with a straight turn and fix the end with a safety pin or adhesive tape. Check that the skin colour above and below the bandage is the same on both limbs. A change of colour indicates the bandage is too tight and should be loosened.

TUBULAR GAUZE FOR TOES AND FINGERS

Tubular gauze is a seamless, tube-shaped bandage, which is easier to apply to fingers and toes than a roller bandage. It comes with an applicator to fix the bandage in place.

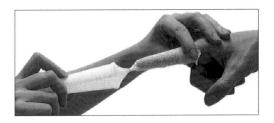

1 Cut a piece of gauze three times longer than the injured finger, and push the whole cut length onto the applicator. Slide the applicator gently over the finger.

2 Hold the end of the gauze firmly onto the base of the finger and gently pull back the applicator, leaving a gauze layer on the finger. Twist the applicator twice, then gently push it back over the finger.

3 With a second layer of gauze in place, withdraw the empty applicator. Fix the gauze in place at the base of the finger or toe with small sections of adhesive tape. Do not encircle the finger with the tape, as this could cut off the blood supply.

ELEVATION SLING

An elevation sling is used to keep the hand and fingers in a raised position and also to provide support for a chest injury or fractured collarbone.

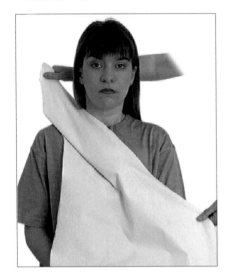

2 Tuck the base of the bandage under the injured arm. Take the lower end up the back to the shoulder. Secure the fingers inside the sling by twisting the end gently before tying the ends at the shoulder.

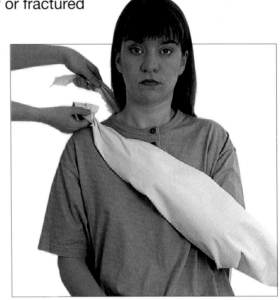

1 Ask the victim to support the injured arm across the chest, with the fingertips touching the opposite shoulder. Hold a triangular bandage over the injured arm, with the longest side over the uninjured side of the body and the point of the triangle over the elbow on the injured side. Wrap the top end of the bandage around the upper hand.

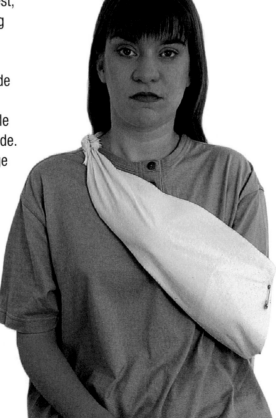

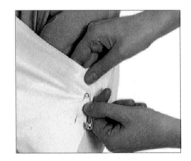

3 At the elbow, ease the loose fabric backwards and tuck the point into the sling, or use a safety pin to secure it. Insert the pin with the point facing downwards for safety. Check the colour of the fingers. If there is any change of colour, a sign of possible impaired circulation, remove the sling and loosen any bandages.

ARM SLING

An arm sling is designed to support the lower arm, hand and fingers across the chest. It is used for various injuries to the upper or lower arm and wrist, including some fractures.

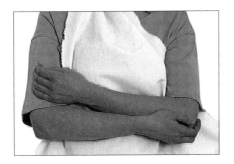

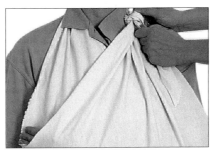

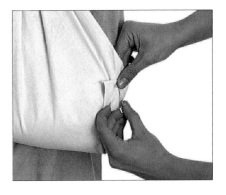

1 Ask the victim to support the injured arm as shown above. Hold the longest side of the sling down the uninjured side of the body, with the top end around the back of the neck.

2 Bring the lower end of bandage up to support the forearm and tie it securely to the other end. The knot should sit in the hollow above the collarbone on the injured side.

3 Bring the point forwards, over the elbow, and fasten it to the front of the sling with a safety pin. Make sure the point faces downwards in case the pin becomes unfastened. Check that hand and wrist are supported in a position that is slightly higher than the elbow.

COLLAR AND CUFF SLING

A collar and cuff sling is used to support an upper arm injury or collarbone fracture, or when the hand and fingers need to be raised. It is also used when an elevation sling would be too uncomfortable for the victim. Before the sling is put in place, make a 'clove hitch' as shown below.

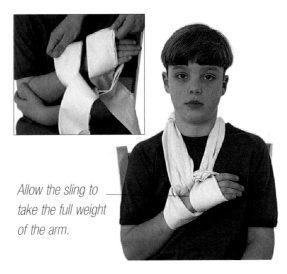

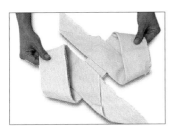

1 For a 'clove hitch', use a triangular bandage folded into a narrow strip. First make two loops, one pointing upwards and one downwards.

Allow the sling to take the full weight of the arm.

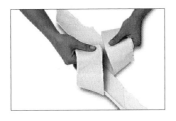

2 Fold both loops into the middle, so that they form a secure and firm support for the arm.

3 Place the injured arm against the chest and in a raised position, with the fingers pointing towards the opposite shoulder. Slip the two loops gently over the hand and place them so that the arm is comfortable and there is no pressure on an injured area.

Bites and stings animal

Take action if any of the following occurs:

- You know someone has been bitten by an animal, or another person

- There is bleeding from a wound made by a bite

- There are teeth marks anywhere that the skin is broken

As well as causing wounds to the skin and deeper tissues, there is a high risk of infection from both animal and human bites unless prompt medical treatment is given. A tetanus injection and antibiotics may be prescribed.

✚ **SEEK URGENT MEDICAL HELP IF AN ANIMAL OR HUMAN BITE HAS BROKEN THE SKIN.**

FOR A SMALL WOUND

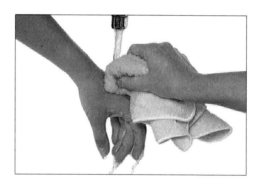

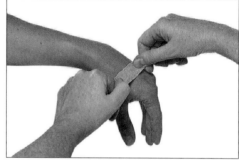

1 Wash the area which has been bitten as thoroughly as possible, using an antiseptic wash or soap and warm water.

2 Dry the area with a clean towel or blot it dry with clean tissues. Apply a sterile adhesive dressing over the entire area of the wound.

FOR A LARGE WOUND

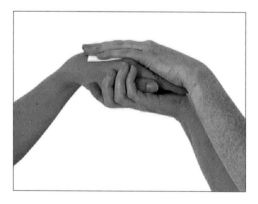

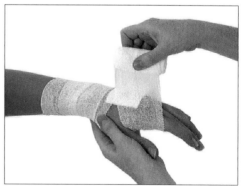

1 Where there is obvious skin damage and some bleeding, apply pressure with your hand or fingers over a sterile or clean dressing. Raise the affected part if possible.

2 When the bleeding is under control, apply a bandage to maintain pressure and keep the dressing in place. Always roll bandages from the inside of the limb outwards.

Bites and stings insect

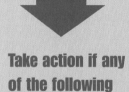

Take action if any of the following occurs:

- Pain, swelling or soreness
- A sting remaining in the skin
- Difficulty in breathing

What to look for:

- Spreading redness and swelling of the skin
- Wheezing or gasping for air
- Rapid pulse

Insect stings may be painful but are usually not serious. A few people are allergic to stings and may develop breathing difficulties with a dramatic fall in blood pressure (anaphylactic shock). Emergency treatment is vital.

✚ **CALL AN AMBULANCE IMMEDIATELY IF THERE ARE SIGNS OF ALLERGY, IF BREATHING DIFFICULTIES DEVELOP, OR IF THE VICTIM HAS MULTIPLE STINGS OR STINGS NEAR THE MOUTH.**

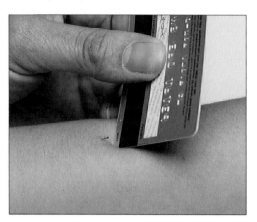

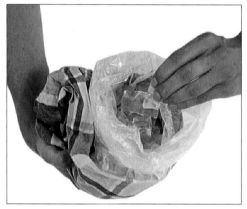

1 If the sting is still in the skin, scrape it out with a fingernail or hard object, such as the corner of a credit card. Do not remove it with tweezers, because this may squeeze more poison into the skin.

2 To relieve pain, prepare a cold compress or an ice pack. Soak a cloth in very cold water and then wring it out, or make an icepack by placing ice cubes in a plastic bag and covering with a damp cloth.

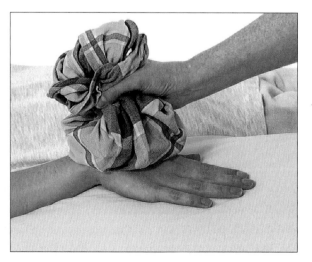

3 Apply the ice pack or cold compress to the site of the sting. An ice pack should not be applied for more than ten minutes every hour, but can be reapplied hourly to relieve pain if needed.

Bleeding internal

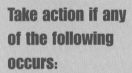

Take action if any of the following occurs:

- Violent injury
- Pain or tenderness
- Bleeding from orifices
- Increasing thirst
- Pattern bruising at the site of injury

What to look for:

- Cold, clammy and pale skin
- Weak and increasingly rapid pulse
- Confusion or irritability
- Collapse or unconsciousness

Internal bleeding means loss of blood into the skull, chest or abdomen. It may follow an injury or be the result of a medical condition, and always requires urgent medical attention. You should suspect internal bleeding if signs of shock (see page 85) develop after an injury with no visible bleeding, or if there is bleeding or fluid loss from body orifices (see table below).

Visible signs of internal bleeding

Body part	Injury	Result
Ear	Fractured skull Damage to ear canal or eardrum	Blood or clear fluid
Nose	Fractured skull Damage to nose	Blood or clear fluid
Mouth	Fractured jaw or damage to mouth	Fresh blood
Lung	Lung or upper airway injury	Bright red frothy blood, coughed up
Stomach	Stomach or duodenal ulcer	Red or dark brown material, like coffee grounds, vomited up
Bowel	Damage to intestines	Fresh blood or black tarry stools
Vagina	Miscarriage Injury to womb or vagina	Fresh or dark blood
Urethra	Damaged kidney, ureter or bladder	Red or smoky urine; blood or clots in urine

1 Help the victim to lie down in the most comfortable position. The victim will choose the position which eases the pain and you should try to provide support for the chosen position with pillows or blankets. Generally, a conscious victim will feel better with the legs raised slightly and this will also help to reduce the symptoms of shock.

✚ CALL AN AMBULANCE AS SOON AS POSSIBLE BECAUSE THE VICTIM MAY SUDDENLY COLLAPSE OR BECOME UNCONSCIOUS.

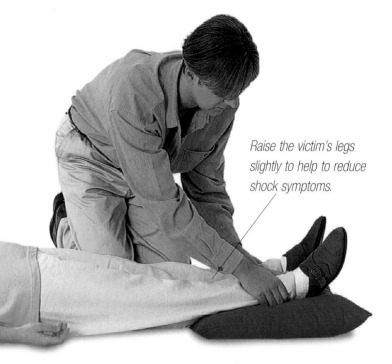

Raise the victim's legs slightly to help to reduce shock symptoms.

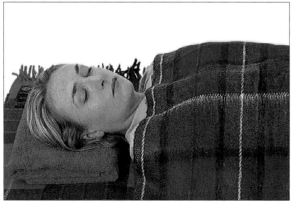

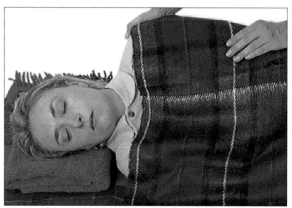

2 Cover the victim lightly with clothing or a blanket. If you are outdoors, ease some fabric, such as a blanket, clothing or even newspapers, under the victim to reduce heat loss from a cold surface. Try to reduce all movement of the victim to avoid further internal blood loss.

3 Reassure the victim at frequent intervals. Keep checking pulse and breathing and monitor for signs of shock (see page 85). Be prepared to start resuscitation if necessary (see page 10). Place an unconscious victim in the recovery position (see page 11).

Bleeding wounds

Take action if the following occurs:

- Bleeding is severe. No time should be lost in applying pressure to reduce the blood loss. Place a clean pad or fabric barrier over the wound, whenever possible, to avoid contact with another person's blood

In the case of a small cut, instinct usually takes over and the victim applies firm pressure over the wound to stop the bleeding and ease the pain. Raising the injured part as high as possible further eases the pain by reducing pressure in the cut blood vessels. The first aid treatment required for severe or deep wounds is exactly the same.

Raise the injured part above the level of the heart to reduce blood flow to the wound.

1 As long as there are no protruding objects, apply direct pressure over the wound, using a sterile dressing or clean pad. If you do not have one, a bulky pad can be made from tissues. Ideally, the victim should apply pressure to his or her own wound, as he or she will know exactly how much to apply.

2 Raise the injured part above the level of the victim's heart. Ask the victim to lie down.

Bandage the dressing in place firmly, but not too tightly.

3 Fix the dressing firmly in position with a clean bandage. If blood seeps through, leave the first dressing in place and apply another bandage on top.

Foreign objects

Seek medical advice as soon as possible. Any foreign object embedded in a wound should be left in place until medical help arrives, so that it can be expertly removed without the risk of causing further damage.

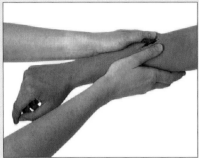

1 If there is a foreign object such as a glass or metal fragment or a large splinter in the wound, apply pressure equally on both sides of the object to stop any bleeding.

2 Build up padding either around, or on both sides of the wound. DO NOT try to remove the foreign object, because this could make any bleeding worse.

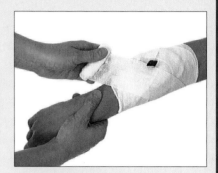

3 Maintain the padding in position with a bandage wrapped in a figure-of-eight (criss-cross) formation around the foreign object.

4 Check fingertip colour to make sure that the bandage is not too tight. If the skin on the injured side looks blue, white or mottled, loosen the bandage. Elevate the wounded area to reduce blood loss.

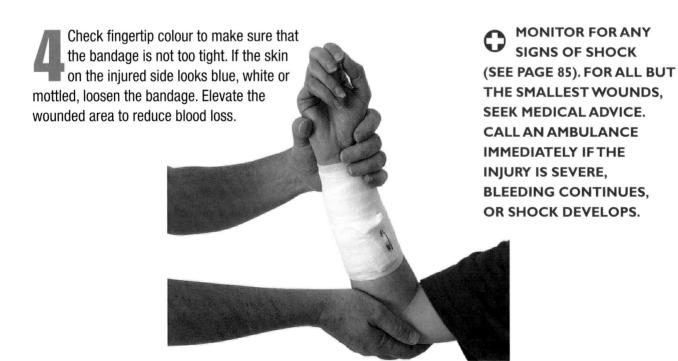

✚ **MONITOR FOR ANY SIGNS OF SHOCK (SEE PAGE 85). FOR ALL BUT THE SMALLEST WOUNDS, SEEK MEDICAL ADVICE. CALL AN AMBULANCE IMMEDIATELY IF THE INJURY IS SEVERE, BLEEDING CONTINUES, OR SHOCK DEVELOPS.**

Bleeding wounds

DEEP CUTS

A deep cut may not appear to be large, but blood vessels, nerves, tendons, ligaments and muscles may have been damaged. If the wound was caused by a long blade, assume there is some internal damage. Most deep wounds need prompt control of bleeding and medical assessment, because of the risk of complications, including tetanus infection.

1 Apply firm pressure over the wound with a sterile dressing to control bleeding. Depending on the location of the injury, either the victim or the first aider can do this. If a sterile dressing is not available, folded tissues may be used.

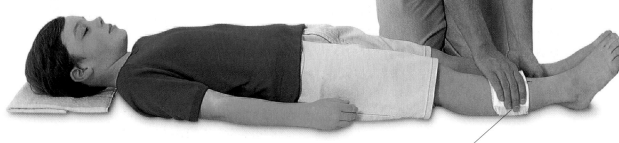

Ensure that bleeding is controlled before preparing to bandage the wound.

✚ **CALL AN AMBULANCE AS SOON AS POSSIBLE.**

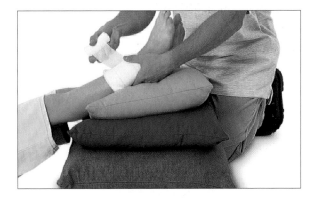

2 Ask the victim to lie down. Raise an injured limb above the level of the heart to reduce blood flow to the part. If an object is protruding from the wound, pad around it before applying a dressing (see page 35). Fix the dressing firmly in position with a bandage.

3 If blood seeps through the dressing, place another one on top. For leg wounds, compare the colour of the toes on both feet and loosen the bandage if the toes on the injured leg start to swell or become discoloured. Treat for shock as necessary.

SURFACE CUTS

Small surface cuts are common. If there is very little bleeding they can usually be treated successfully without any specialist care. However, if the cut is on the face, there is a risk of scarring; if it is on a hand, or if it is deep or gaping, there is a risk of injury to deeper tissues. In these cases, medical advice should be sought.

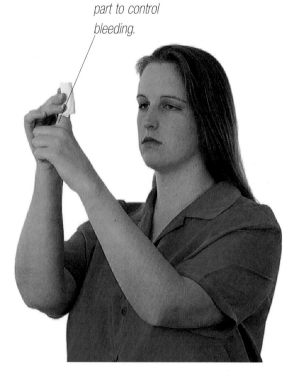

Raise the injured part to control bleeding.

1 Control any bleeding by applying firm pressure over the wound. The victim should hold either a sterile dressing or one or two folded tissues firmly over the wound. Raise the injured part as high as possible to reduce blood flow to the area.

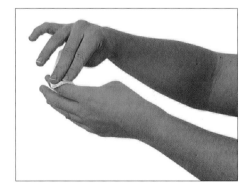

2 Clean the wound thoroughly with either an antiseptic solution or soap and warm water. Use a gauze or cotton swab and wipe away from the wound to avoid soiling it with any skin bacteria. Use several swabs if necessary, using each one once only.

✚ **IF BLEEDING CONTINUES, SEEK MEDICAL ADVICE PROMPTLY.**

● **IF THE WOUND HAS NOT PARTIALLY HEALED WITHIN 24 HOURS, SEEK MEDICAL ADVICE.**

3 Apply an adhesive dressing. Advise the victim to remove the dressing at night to allow the wound to dry. A new adhesive dressing should only be applied if the wound is moist and appears to need protection.

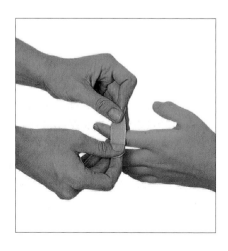

Blisters

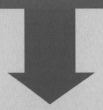

Take action if any of the following occurs:

- Severe pain, or no pain but loss of sensation
- Hot, sensitive skin

What to look for:

- Black or red skin which may be blistered
- Swelling
- Clear fluid weeping from the skin

Blisters form as a result of allergic reaction, infection, friction or heat. They are caused by fluid leaking into a damaged or infected area under the skin's surface. This creates a protective cushion which allows new skin to form below the blister. If there is a risk that a blister could be damaged by friction, it should be protected by a dressing. Never burst a blister, as this can cause infection.

Identifying types of blister

Cause	Symptom	Action
Injury 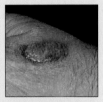	Injury is visible and with obvious cause such as friction, heat, chemical burns or insect bites. Blisters are usually more than 5mm (¼in) in diameter.	Do not burst a blister; cover it with a dry dressing. Seek medical advice promptly if redness spreads out from the blister and pain increases, as infection is possible.
Cold sore (herpes simplex) 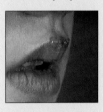	A crop of blisters in one area, usually on or around the mouth and less than 5mm (¼in) in diameter. Blisters are preceded by skin tingling and pain.	Apply an antiviral cream as soon as possible. Seek medical advice urgently if the rash spreads beyond the original outbreak.
Shingles (herpes zoster) 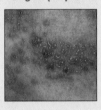	Blisters are usually less than 5mm (¼in) in diameter. They always occur on one side of the body, spreading out in a band around the trunk or down a limb.	Seek medical advice urgently as shingles is contagious: avoid contact with adults who have not had chickenpox, especially pregnant women, until the last blister has burst and scabbed over.
Eczema 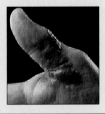	Blisters are often more than 5mm (¼in) in diameter, and may be painful. Commonly appear on hands, palms or soles of feet.	Seek medical advice as soon as possible, urgently if the skin is very painful – this is unusual and may indicate that the skin is infected.

Bruises

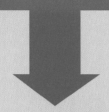

Take action if any of the following occurs:

- Pain at the injury site
- Pressure builds up beneath the skin

What to look for:

- A blueish discoloration around the site of the injury
- Swelling of the injured area

Bruises are caused by a blunt blow to the skin, which breaks the tiny blood vessels, or capillaries, close to the surface, so that blood seeps into the tissues. Sometimes there is a more serious underlying injury. The colour of a bruise gradually changes as the blood is reabsorbed into the body.

If the injury is only a few minutes old, first reduce the spread of bleeding into the tissues by raising the affected part and applying an ice pack or cold compress (see page 31). This helps to lessen any later pain and swelling. After ten minutes of firm pressure, treat any associated injuries, such as a sprain (see pages 86–87).

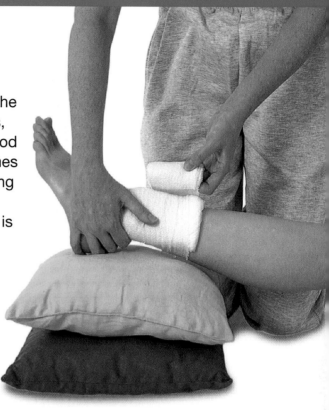

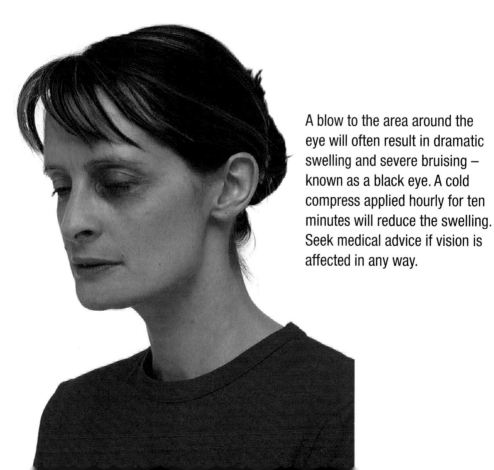

A blow to the area around the eye will often result in dramatic swelling and severe bruising – known as a black eye. A cold compress applied hourly for ten minutes will reduce the swelling. Seek medical advice if vision is affected in any way.

Burns and scalds

Take action if any of the following occurs:

- Severe pain or no pain (see right)
- Cold, clammy skin
- Nausea or vomiting

What to look for:

- Black or red skin which may be blistered
- Swelling
- Clear fluid weeping from the skin

Burns are caused by contact with a heat source such as hot metal, or by corrosive chemicals, friction, radiation or electricity. Scalds are caused by steam or hot liquid. The amount of pain felt is not a true guide to the severity of the injury. Superficial and partial-thickness burns (involving only the skin) have a tendency to be more painful than full-thickness burns, in which the underlying tissues are damaged and nerve endings are destroyed.

✚ **DO NOT BURST ANY BLISTERS THAT FORM AFTER A BURN OR SCALD.**

1 Cool the burn or scald at once with cold running water from the nearest tap. In an emergency, any cold, non-flammable fluid can be used. Continue cooling with cold water for at least ten minutes, even if the burn has stopped hurting. Do not apply any lotion, ointment or oil to a burn or scald.

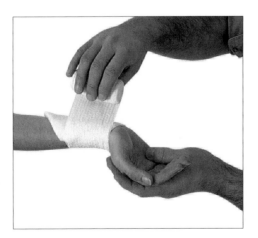

✚ **SEEK MEDICAL HELP FOR ALL BUT THE MOST MINOR BURN. IF THE BURN IS DEEP OR COVERS AN AREA GREATER THAN THE SIZE OF THE VICTIM'S OWN PALM, CALL AN AMBULANCE.**

2 Remove any jewellery from the burned area in case of swelling. Cover the burn with a clean, non-stick dressing to reduce the risk of infection.

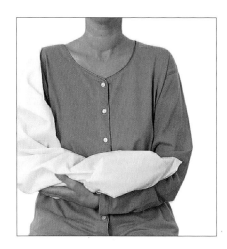

3 Do not try to remove clothing or debris stuck to the burn, since this could increase the risk of infection. Cut around any attached material and cover the burned area. If a sterile dressing is not available, use a clean plastic bag, plastic film, or any clean, non-fluffy material.

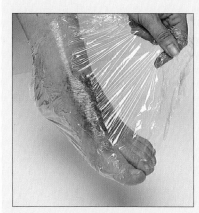

If a sterile dressing is not available, use plastic film or a plastic bag.

4 While waiting for help, keep monitoring the victim's pulse and breathing and check for signs of shock (see page 85). Be prepared to resuscitate if necessary. Avoid giving any food or drink, unless the burn is very small, in case an anaesthetic may be needed. Monitor the victim's breathing, especially after smoke inhalation, and be prepared to give CPR (cardiopulmonary resuscitation, see page 13) if necessary.

Raise the legs on a blanket or pillow.

Treatment of burns and scalds

Chemical burn

First, make the area safe. Flood the burnt part with water for at least 20 minutes (longer than for a heat burn). Meanwhile, call an ambulance and monitor breathing – be prepared to resuscitate the victim if necessary (see page 10). Gently remove any contaminated clothing. Send details of the chemical involved with the victim to hospital.

Electrical burn

Electricity, including a lightning strike, leaves burns both where the current entered and where it left the body. There is also a high risk of cardiac arrest. Make sure that the power source is safe before approaching the victim. Call an ambulance immediately, then treat burn injuries by cooling while waiting for help. If cardiac arrest occurs, give CPR (cardiopulmonary resuscitation, see page 13) until the ambulance arrives.

Burns to the airway

Burns to the face, or inhalation of smoke in a fire, can be very dangerous. The victim may suffer pain and extensive swelling of the lining of the mouth and throat, resulting in the narrowing or closure of the upper airway. This can be life-threatening. Call an ambulance at once if you know the victim has inhaled smoke or if you notice soot or damaged skin around the mouth or nose, swelling of the mouth or tongue, or breathing difficulties. Observe the victim closely in case resuscitation is needed.

Chest injuries

Take action if any of the following occurs:

- Difficulty breathing, with shallow and gasping breaths
- Chest pain

What to look for:

- Bright red, frothy blood coughed up
- Blueness of tongue and lips
- Sucking noise as air enters the chest cavity with each breath
- Bloodstained fluid bubbling around the wound

An injury to the chest can cause internal bleeding or lung damage, which may be life-threatening.

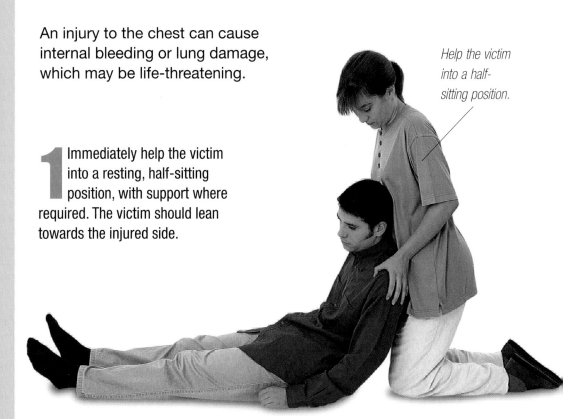

Help the victim into a half-sitting position.

1 Immediately help the victim into a resting, half-sitting position, with support where required. The victim should lean towards the injured side.

✚ **CALL FOR AN AMBULANCE AS SOON AS POSSIBLE.**

2 Check for a penetrating wound. If one is found, place a thick, sterile dressing or pad of clean tissues over the wound and press down gently but firmly with the palm of your hand. This should stop any bleeding and restrict the entry of air into the chest cavity.

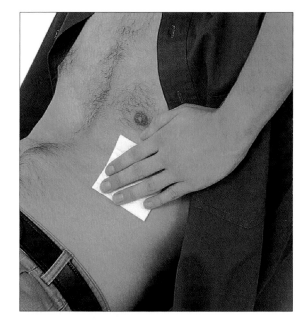

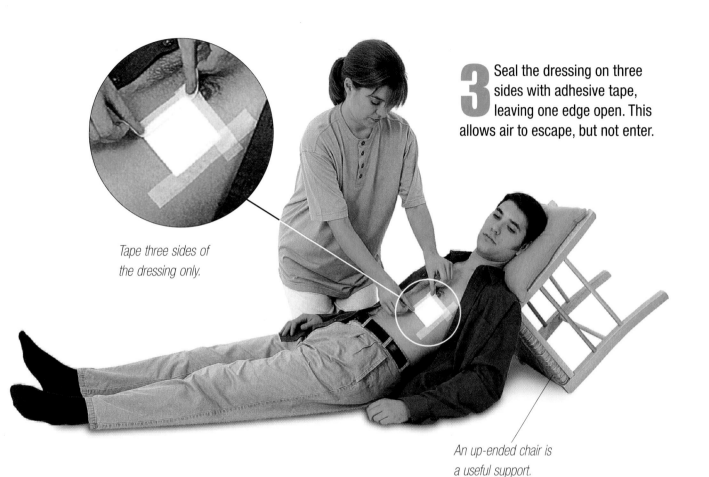

3 Seal the dressing on three sides with adhesive tape, leaving one edge open. This allows air to escape, but not enter.

Tape three sides of the dressing only.

An up-ended chair is a useful support.

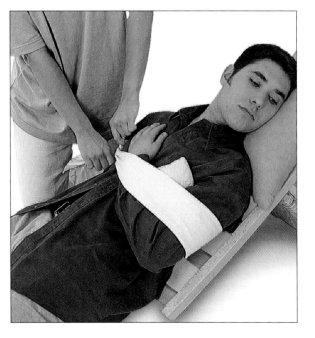

4 Place some padding over the dressing, between the arm and chest wall. Then apply a broad bandage around the chest and over the arm on the injured side to provide support to the injured area.

5 Monitor breathing and pulse while awaiting the ambulance. If the victim becomes unconscious, be prepared to give CPR (cardiopulmonary resuscitation, see page 13). Place the victim in the recovery position but with the injured side downwards. This allows the uninjured lung to work efficiently.

Childbirth

When a baby arrives unexpectedly but after a normal pregnancy, he or she will usually be born naturally, without any complications. Labour has three stages: first, the birth canal stretches and the uterus contracts every few minutes in preparation for pushing the baby out – this may last for several hours, with contractions gradually increasing in frequency and intensity; second, the baby is born; third, the placenta (afterbirth) is delivered. There is usually plenty of time to arrange assistance. If not, stay calm and listen to the mother's wishes. Never try to delay the birth, and interfere as little as possible – the baby will usually be expelled naturally. DO NOT pull on the head and shoulders as they emerge.

1 Help the mother to assume whatever position is most comfortable for her. Provide support if she wishes with pillows or rolled-up clothing. Place clean towels or old cotton sheeting under her for the birth.

2 Wash your hands and scrub under the nails throroughly, if there is time, and wear plastic gloves if available. Encourage the mother to rest between contractions. When the birth is imminent, the widest part of the baby's head will become visible. At this stage, ask the mother to stop pushing, and take fast, short breaths instead.

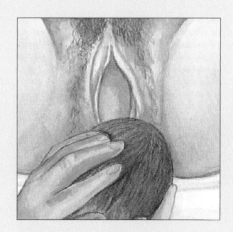

3 When the baby's head appears,support it lightly on your hands until the next contraction comes and expels the body. The head will rotate slightly on your hands as the shoulders turn sideways ready to be born. Do not interfere with the natural movement of the baby because any resistance can be harmful.

✚ **CALL FOR MEDICAL ASSISTANCE AS SOON AS POSSIBLE.**

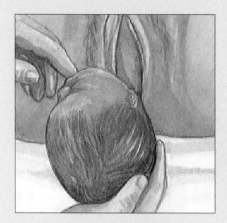

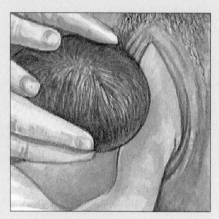

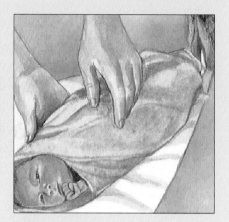

4 If there is any membrane covering the face, gently remove it to enable the baby to breathe. Check to see if a loop of cord is around the baby's neck. If so, carefully slip it over the head to avoid it tightening around the neck as the baby is born.

5 At the start of the next contraction, the shoulders will appear, one at a time. Do not attempt to pull on the baby but let the mother's contractions do the work naturally.

6 When the baby slips out of the birth canal, lift it away carefully – it will be slippery. Gently pass the baby to the mother and place it on her abdomen.

7 Cover the baby in a towel or blanket to maintain warmth, keeping the head covered to conserve heat. Keep the head low so that fluid and mucous can drain from the mouth. DO NOT pull on or cut the umbilical cord.

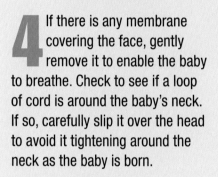

IF THE BABY DOES NOT BREATHE ON ITS OWN, IMMEDIATELY CHECK THE AIRWAY (SEE PAGES 8–9) AND BE PREPARED TO CARRY OUT RESUSCITATION (SEE PAGE 10). DO NOT SMACK THE BABY.

8 A short time after the birth, the placenta (afterbirth) will be expelled. This will happen naturally with the mother's contractions – DO NOT pull on the cord. Wrap the placenta in a plastic bag, but leave it still attached to the baby. The midwife will want to examine it, to ensure that there are no fragments left inside the mother, which could be dangerous. Leave it to the midwife to cut the cord.

9 It is normal for the mother to bleed a little after the birth. If available, supply warm water and towels and help her to clean herself up. Provide a sanitary towel if available.

✚ **IF BLEEDING IS SEVERE, WATCH FOR SIGNS OF SHOCK (SEE PAGE 85) AND CALL AN AMBULANCE, IF ONE IS NOT ALREADY ON ITS WAY.**

Choking

Take action if any of the following occurs:

- Difficulty in breathing (shortness of breath)
- Difficulty in speaking

What to look for:

- Clutching the throat
- Distress
- Noisy breathing, wheezing or a high-pitched 'crowing' noise
- Inability to speak
- Congested facial skin with blueish lips
- Later, collapse and unconsciousness

In a choking emergency, it is vital to determine whether the victim is moving any air in and out of the lungs. If there is total obstruction of the airway, the victim will quickly collapse. In a partial airway blockage there is time to get medical aid before collapse is likely.

1 Be reassuring and encourage coughing. DO NOT slap the person on the back – this can push objects farther down the airway. Don't let a choking person rush from the room in embarrassment.

➕ **CHOKING CAN CAUSE DEATH WITHIN MINUTES – TREAT IT AS AN EMERGENCY.**

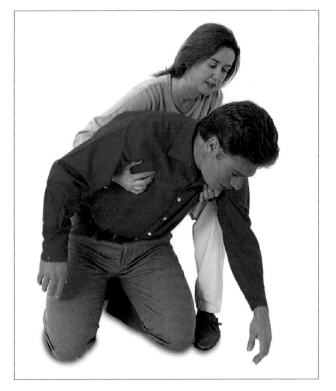

2 Help the person to bend forwards so the head is lower than the chest. Check inside the mouth and remove any obvious obstruction.

If the victim becomes unconscious

1 Call an ambulance as a first priority or ask someone else to do this.

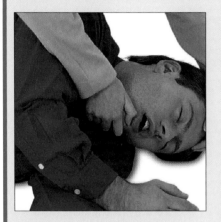

2 Attempt to clear any obstruction from the person's mouth.

3 Give abdominal thrusts by rolling the victim onto the back and kneeling astride him or her. Place the heel of one hand mid-way between the navel and breastbone, cover it with the other hand and keep your elbows straight (as for CPR). Press sharply upwards and inwards several times. Check the mouth again.

4 If the airway is apparently clear and breathing is still absent, begin resuscitation (see page 10) in an attempt to blow air past the obstruction.

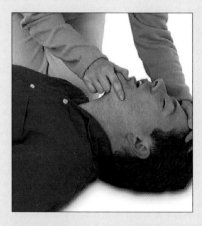

5 Check for breathing and circulation. Start CPR (cardiopulmonary resuscitation, see page 13), if necessary. Repeat abdominal thrusts in-between each CPR cycle if necessary.

3 If this fails, perform the Heimlich or abdominal thrust manoeuvre. Stand behind the person and place one clenched fist, thumb inwards, just below the breastbone. Grasp this fist with your other hand and pull sharply upwards and inwards. The object should shoot out as air is forced violently outwards. Repeat up to five times if necessary, then check inside the mouth again.

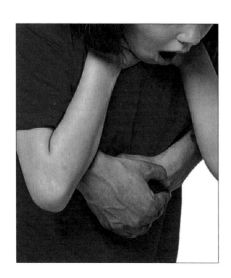

✚ **NEVER PRACTISE THE HEIMLICH MANOEUVRE ON ANYONE WHO ISN'T CHOKING – THERE IS A RISK OF DAMAGE TO THE INTERNAL ORGANS.**

Choking child

Toddlers and older children

1 Encourage the child to bend forwards and cough, to clear any obstructions from the mouth.

2 Stand behind the child and place a clenched fist against the lower breastbone. Grasp with the other hand and give up to five chest thrusts by pulling sharply upwards and inwards. Check the mouth.

3 If this fails, place your fist on the upper abdomen and perform the Heimlich manoeuvre, as for adults (see page 47).

4 If the child lapses into unconsciousness, start CPR (cardiopulmonary resuscitation, see page 13).

For a baby

1 Lay the baby face down over your forearm with the head lower than the chest.

2 Give up to five sharp back slaps between the shoulder blades to dislodge any obstruction.

3 Check the mouth and remove any obvious obstruction.

4 If this fails, place the baby face upwards and put two fingertips onto the lower part of the breastbone, just below the nipples. Press vigorously up to five times and check the mouth again.

✚ **DO NOT USE ABDOMINAL THRUSTS ON A BABY.**

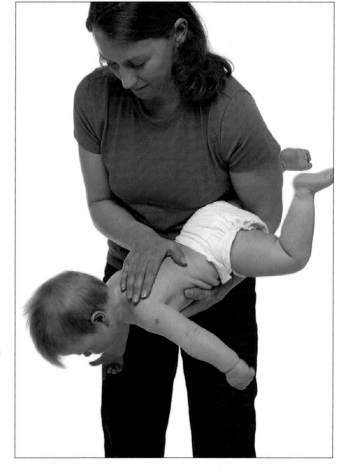

Collarbone fracture

Take action if any
of the following
occurs:

- Pain and tenderness at or around the injury site
- Pain increased by even slight movement
- Nausea or vomiting

What to look for:

- The victim supporting the weight of the arm at the elbow
- Head tilted to the injured side to ease the pain
- Injured shoulder joint a little lower than the uninjured side
- Obvious swelling or deformity over the injury site
- A reluctance to move any part of the trunk or injured limb

The collarbone, which runs between the shoulder blade and breastbone, is usually broken by a blow to the shoulder or by a fall onto the outstretched hand.

1 Ask the victim to sit down and support the injured limb at the elbow with the other hand. The injured shoulder often droops lower than the uninjured side because the shoulder joint has lost the support of the collarbone.

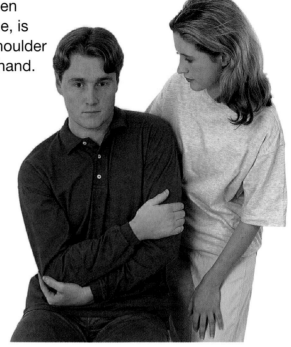

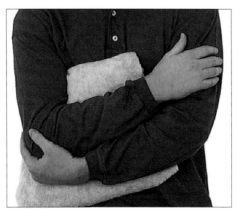

2 Gently ease soft padding – such as a folded towel or sweater – between the arm and chest wall to provide extra support.

3 Support the injured arm with an elevation sling (see page 28).

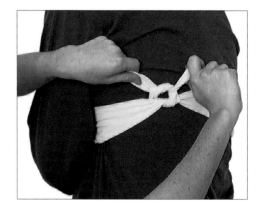

4 Apply a broad bandage around the body, fastening the arm against the chest. Tie off using a secure knot on the uninjured side of the body.

✚ **SEEK MEDICAL ADVICE PROMPTLY, IF A FRACTURE IS SUSPECTED.**

Concussion

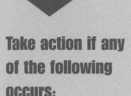

Take action if any of the following occurs:

- Headache
- Nausea or vomiting
- Tiredness
- Blurred or double vision

What to look for:

- Temporary loss of consciousness
- Confusion or disorientation
- Irritability
- Loss of hand-to-eye coordination
- Short-term memory loss of events before the accident

Concussion is a head injury which can follow a blow to the head or jaw, or result from a heavy fall onto the head, feet or buttocks. The jarring that occurs causes the brain to be shaken around inside the skull, causing internal bruising, swelling and sometimes bleeding. Sometimes, a brief loss of consciousness occurs with concussion.

➕ **CALL FOR AN AMBULANCE, AND WATCH FOR ANY CHANGE IN THE VICTIM'S CONDITION WHILE YOU WAIT.**

1 Check the victim's response to simple instructions such as, 'Squeeze my hand. Now let it go'. If the victim fails to respond promptly, turn them onto their side immediately because they may lose consciousness.

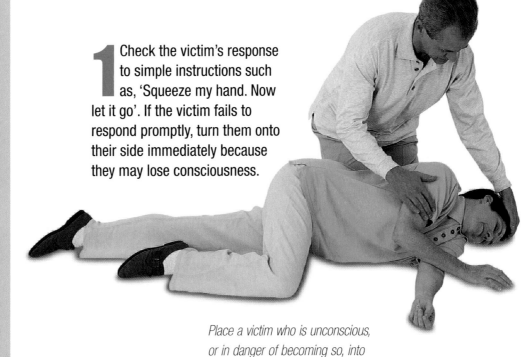

Place a victim who is unconscious, or in danger of becoming so, into the recovery position (see page 11).

2 If the victim is fully conscious, help them into a comfortable position, preferably with the head slightly raised. Check for any injuries, including wounds, bumps or bruises. If a wound is found, stop any bleeding promptly with direct pressure, elevation and rest for the injured part.

3 If there is a bump or bruise on the head, prepare a cold compress (see page 31) and encourage the victim to hold it in place so that you can check their ability to coordinate the task. Observe the victim closely for any deterioration, including sleepiness, irritability or headache.

Convulsion

Child convulsions usually occur before the age of five years and are not related to epilepsy. During a convulsion, the body will twitch and jerk. These movements are caused by an overheated brain, which results from a high temperature or the start of an infection. The convulsion usually lasts no more than two minutes, often less. Doctors no longer recommend active cooling of a feverish child because this makes the fever recur.

Take action if any of the following occurs:

- Twitching or jerking movements of the trunk and limbs
- Unconsciousness: no response to voice or to touch

What to look for:

- Flushed, ill appearance
- High temperature of 38°C (100°F) or more
- Skin hot to the touch with blueish lips

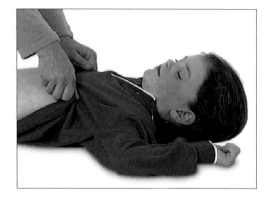

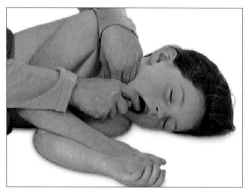

1 Remove all clothing, including any bedclothes, to allow the child to cool down naturally, but do not sponge with water or fan the child's skin.

2 Move the child into the bathroom and run the hot tap to create a steamy atmosphere. This will help to relieve the swelling and inflammation in the upper airways.

3 When the convulsions have stopped, check the child's pulse and breathing and cover him or her with a light sheet or a thin blanket. Repeat the pulse checks every 10–15 minutes, until the child has recovered fully.

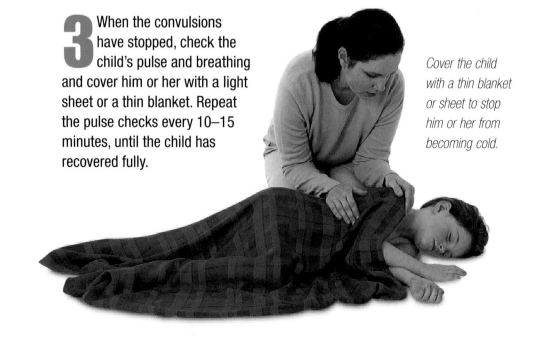

Cover the child with a thin blanket or sheet to stop him or her from becoming cold.

Cramp

Take action if any of the following occurs:

- Waking at night due to muscle spasm
- Chest pain

Keeping a limb in one position for a long time can slow the circulation to major muscles in one area of the body, causing a tight muscle mass in the affected area and cramp. In hot weather, cramps occur when the victim has failed to maintain an adequate fluid intake. A cramp may also occur in cold conditions or following heavy exercise.

Lower leg

Help the victim to lie down and slowly straighten the affected leg while gently pressing down on the knee with your other hand. Hold the foot under the heel and use the other hand to gently push the toes upwards. When the spasm eases, gently massage the affected muscles until the area feels relaxed.

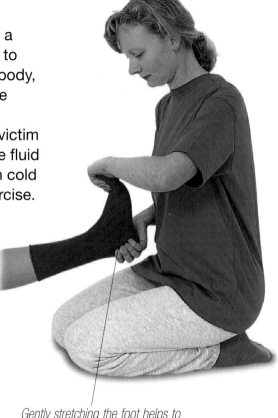

Gently stretching the foot helps to relieve lower leg cramp.

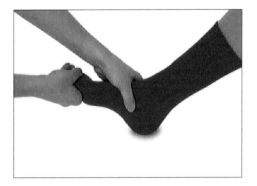

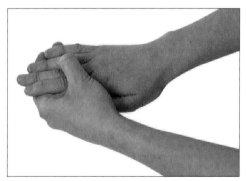

Foot

Ask the victim to stand with the affected foot firmly on the floor. If the toes are in severe spasm, gently try to straighten them with your hand. In cold weather, advise the victim to put on some warm socks.

Hand

Ask the victim to straighten and massage the affected fingers until the muscles relax. Warmth can be comforting when the spasm eases, especially in cold weather.

Croup

Take action if any of the following occurs:

- A barking or crowing sound with each intake of breath
- Frequent coughing

What to look for:

- Spasms of coughing that cause breathlessness
- Exhaustion from frequent coughing
- Deteriorating skin colour with blueish lips and fingertips
- High temperature of 38°C (100°F) or more
- Attempts to sit upright to make breathing easier

Croup is a breathing disorder that affects babies and small children. The attacks often occur at night and are caused by an infection which leads to swelling of the upper respiratory tract.

1 Help the child to breathe more effectively by propping him or her upright with a pile of pillows. Give plenty of reassurance.

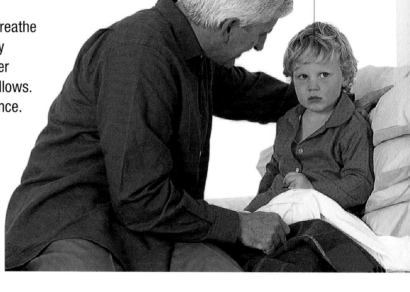

Reassure the child, because croup is a very frightening condition.

2 Create a steamy atmosphere to help to relieve the inflammation and swelling in the upper respiratory tract. Take the child into the bathroom and run the hot tap for some time. For safety, keep the child a safe distance from the tap.

✚ **IF BREATHING DOES NOT IMPROVE RAPIDLY, SEEK MEDICAL HELP PROMPTLY, AS IT MAY BE NECESSARY TO GIVE ANTIBIOTICS.**

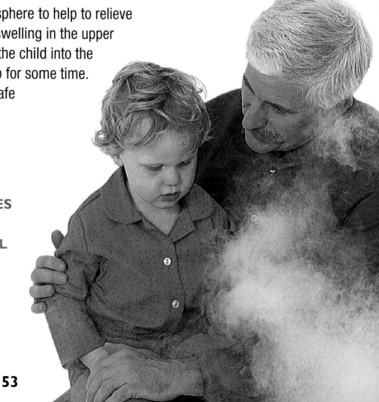

Crush injury

Crush injuries are usually very serious, leading to extensive soft tissue and bone damage. Toxins build up around the injury so that if the crushing force is suddenly removed there is a risk of serious complications from kidney failure.

1 If the casualty has been crushed for less than ten minutes, remove the crushing force, if possible. While waiting for an ambulance, treat any wounds or fractures, and watch for signs of shock (see page 85).

2 If the victim has been crushed for more than ten minutes, DO NOT attempt to remove the crushing force. Offer reassurance and make the victim as comfortable as possible while waiting for the ambulance.

✚ **CALL AN AMBULANCE AS SOON AS POSSIBLE. WHILE WAITING, NOTE ANY CHANGES IN THE VICTIM'S CONDITION.**

Take action if any of the following occurs:

- Tingling or numbness in the affected area
- Feeling cold, faint, dizzy and nauseous
- Severe pain

What to look for:

- Swelling and bruising of the crushed tissues
- Pale, cold and clammy skin
- Signs of a crushing force on the trunk or a limb

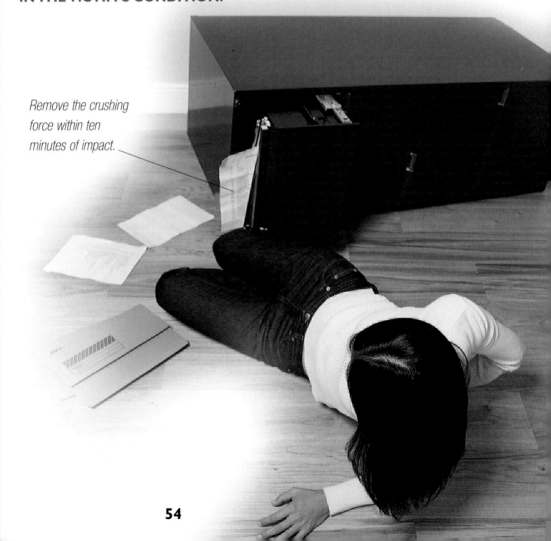

Remove the crushing force within ten minutes of impact.

Cuts, grazes and splinters

Take action if any of the following occurs:

- Pain at the site of injury
- Profuse bleeding
- A splinter in a wound
- Broken skin
- Numbness of the skin
- Deep cuts on a hand or the face
- Difficulty in moving part of a limb or a digit

Minor wounds are very common. A cut may not appear to be serious, but if it is deep or gaping, underlying structures may have been damaged. Cuts on the face may lead to scarring, and cuts on the fingers or hands can cause muscle or tendon damage. Seek prompt medical assessment if you are in any doubt.

Splinters

Splinters are very common. Ensure the area is clean, then remove the splinter with tweezers. If unsuccessful, or if the splinter breaks off, seek medical advice.

Cuts

Make sure your hands are clean, and clean the wound with running water or antiseptic. Apply firm pressure to stop any bleeding. Elevate the wound if bleeding continues. When bleeding stops, apply a sterile dressing, secured with a bandage if necessary.

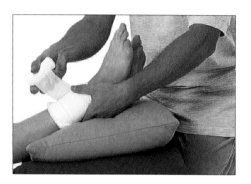

✚ **IF BLEEDING FROM A CUT CONTINUES, SEEK MEDICAL ADVICE PROMPTLY.**

Grazes

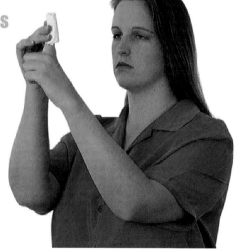

2 Clean the wound thoroughly with an antiseptic or soap and warm water. Use a gauze or cotton swab and wipe away from the wound to avoid soiling it with skin bacteria.

✚ **SEEK MEDICAL ADVICE IF THE WOUND HAS NOT PARTIALLY HEALED WITHIN 24 HOURS.**

1 Control any bleeding by applying firm pressure over the wound using a sterile dressing or tissues and the palm of your hand. Raise the injured part as high as possible to reduce blood flow to the area.

Diabetic complications

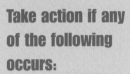

Take action if any of the following occurs:

LOW BLOOD SUGAR

- Feeling faint, giddy and weak with trembling limbs
- Shaking or trembling
- Confusion or strange behaviour in a known diabetic

What to look for:

- Pale skin and sweating
- Confusion or aggressive behaviour
- Shallow breathing with a rapid pulse

HIGH BLOOD SUGAR

- Unconsciousness
- Dry skin and rapid pulse
- Difficult or noisy breathing

What to look for:

- Smell of pear drops or nail-varnish remover on the breath

Diabetes occurs when the body cannot control the level of blood sugar properly, because of a lack of the hormone insulin. Even with treatment, blood sugar levels can become imbalanced, causing problems. The most common emergency for a diabetic is low blood sugar, known medically as hypoglycaemia. Unconsciousness can occur rapidly without emergency treatment. If the victim is suffering from too much sugar, known as hyperglycaemia, deterioration is slower and there is usually plenty of time to call an ambulance.

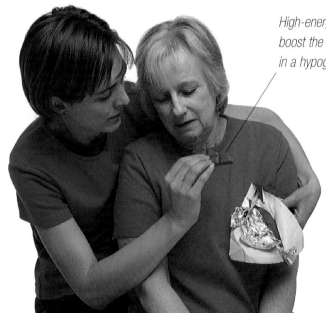

High-energy foods quickly boost the blood sugar levels in a hypoglycaemic attack.

If low blood sugar is suspected, give a conscious victim a sweet drink or sugar lumps to suck, followed by high-energy food such as chocolate, cake, biscuits or a sandwich to raise the blood sugar level.

Place an unconscious victim in the recovery position (see page 11), ensuring that the airway is kept clear. Call an ambulance at once. If necessary, give the person CPR (cardiopulmonary resuscitation, see page 13).

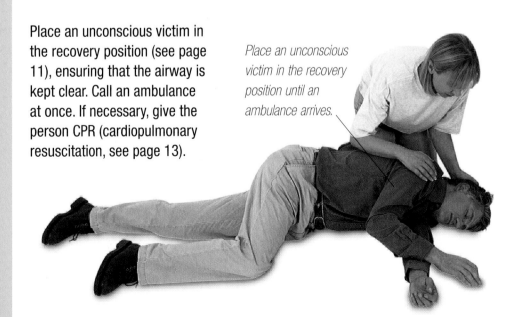

Place an unconscious victim in the recovery position until an ambulance arrives.

Dislocation

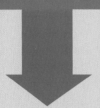

Take action if any of the following occurs:

- An inability to move the injured part
- Severe pain in and around the joint, increased by movement
- Some loss of sensation

What to look for:

- Obvious deformity and swelling around the joint
- Bruising

A dislocation occurs when a severe twist or wrench displaces a bone from its normal position in a joint. There may also be bone fracture and damage to nearby blood vessels and nerves which can cause serious complications.

✚ **TREAT ALL DISLOCATIONS AS FRACTURES UNTIL A DIAGNOSIS IS MADE.**

Elbow

1 Help the victim to find a position in which the injured area can be supported and made more comfortable. A dislocated shoulder, hip or elbow joint can be supported by pillows or blankets. DO NOT try to replace the dislocated bones because this may cause further damage and risk complications.

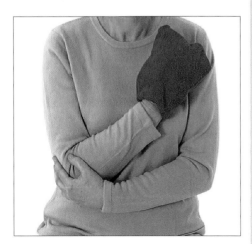

2 For a dislocated finger, use soft padding to support the injury. Wrap a bandage lightly in place unless this is more painful. Do not apply firm pressure because of the risk of further damage to nerves and blood vessels.

Shoulder

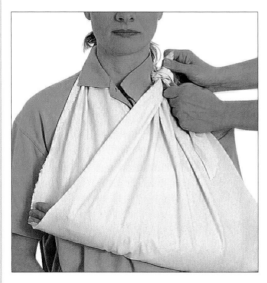

1 For a dislocated finger, place the arm across the chest and support it using a triangular bandage as a sling (see page 28).

✚ **SEEK MEDICAL ADVICE URGENTLY, BECAUSE THERE IS OFTEN A RISK OF COMPLICATIONS. CALL AN AMBULANCE AS SOON AS POSSIBLE IF THE VICTIM IS IN SEVERE PAIN.**

Drowning

Drowning is a common cause of accidental death, especially in children. Summon help immediately – prompt rescue followed by efficient cardiopulmonary resuscitation can save lives. Unless you are a very strong swimmer, you should not enter the water yourself, since this can place your own life at risk.

Take action if any of the following occurs:

- Anyone is struggling in the water
- A victim is lying or floating face-down in the water

What to look for:

- In a rescued person, mottled blue or white skin colour, noisy breathing or no breathing at all and an inability to speak

1 Whenever possible, throw the victim a flotation device, rope, or hold out a pole or tree branch. Unless you are a trained lifesaver, or the victim is unconscious, do not enter the water.

2 If it is necessary to go into the water, wade rather than swim if possible. Attempt rescue from deep water only if you are a strong swimmer. Carry an unconscious victim with the head low, so there is less chance of choking.

3 If the victim is unconscious, check the pulse and be prepared to start cardiopulmonary resuscitation (see page 13). If not, place the victim in the recovery position (see page 11) and continue to check pulse and breathing while awaiting help.

4 Anyone who has been in water for more than a few minutes is at risk of hypothermia (see page 76). Remove wet clothing and cover with towels, blankets or clothing to warm the victim as soon as possible. If the victim regains consciousness, give hot drinks while awaiting help.

Check pulse and breathing and be prepared to resuscitate if necessary.

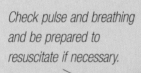

✚ **CALL FOR AN AMBULANCE AS SOON AS POSSIBLE, UNLESS THE VICTIM APPEARS TO BE FULLY RECOVERED. ANYONE RESCUED FROM WATER MUST BE ASSESSED BY A DOCTOR.**

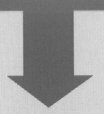

Ear problems

Take action if any of the following occurs:

- Sharp pain
- Bleeding from the ear
- Clear or straw-coloured fluid draining from the ear canal
- Hearing loss
- Persistent earache with fever
- Foreign body wedged in the ear canal

The ears can be damaged by blows to the head, sudden loud noises, pressure waves from an explosion or foreign bodies inserted into the ear canal. Earache is most often due to infection, and commonly occurs during or after a cold or other respiratory infection.

Does the victim have any:
- Bleeding or fluid draining from the ear canal?
- Severe pain in the ear?

NO →

Has the victim experienced:
- Sudden loss of hearing?
- Ringing in the ears?
- Dizziness?
- Foreign body stuck in the ear canal?

YES ↓

SEEK MEDICAL ADVICE URGENTLY

YES ↓

MAKE AN APPOINTMENT WITH A DOCTOR

An insect lodged in the ear canal can usually be removed by flooding the ear with water.

✚ **IF THERE IS NO IMPROVEMENT WITHIN 24 HOURS, SEEK MEDICAL ADVICE PROMPTLY.**

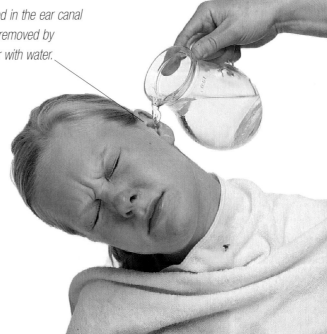

Electric shock

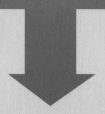

Take action if any of the following occurs:

- Burns at the site of entry and discharge of electric current
- Difficulty breathing
- Collapse and unconsciousness
- No pulse

✚ DO NOT TOUCH THE VICTIM UNTIL THE CURRENT HAS BEEN DISCONNECTED.

LOW-VOLTAGE ELECTRIC SHOCK

Electrical accidents can occur when equipment or household appliances have a fault, such as a damaged flex, or when they are used in an unsafe manner, such as handling an appliance with wet hands.

1 Never touch the victim until you are certain that contact with the electric current has been broken, or you could be electrocuted yourself. Switch off the power, at the mains if possible, then disconnect the appliance from the power point.

✚ CALL AN AMBULANCE IMMEDIATELY.

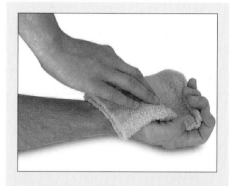

If the skin has been burned, flood with cold water for at least ten minutes, then apply a cold compress (see page 31).

2 If you cannot switch the current off, stand on some insulating material – wood, rubber, plastic or thick paper. Use a wooden pole, not a metal one, to push the current source clear or pull the victim away by a loop of rope if you can, or by tugging on clothing.

3 If the victim is unconscious, start CPR (cardiopulmonary resuscitation, see page 13) if necessary. If the victim is breathing and has a pulse, look for burns on the skin where the electricity entered the body and where it went to earth. Cool any burns with cold water (see page 40). Once the victim is breathing, place him or her in the recovery position (see page 11).

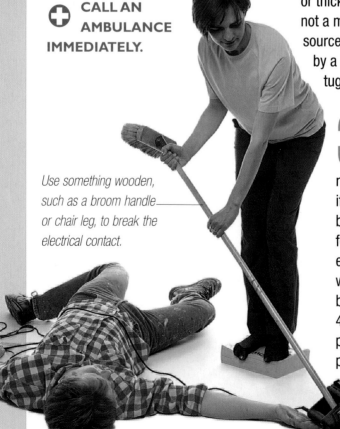

Use something wooden, such as a broom handle or chair leg, to break the electrical contact.

HIGH-VOLTAGE ELECTRIC SHOCK

Power lines and overhead high tension cables have such a high voltage current that contact is usually fatal. The current can arc or jump over a considerable distance and can cause injury to a person from as far away as 18 metres (20 yards). Wood and other insulators are no protection.

1 Call the local electricity supply authority for help, and keep bystanders well clear of the accident until the power has been turned off.

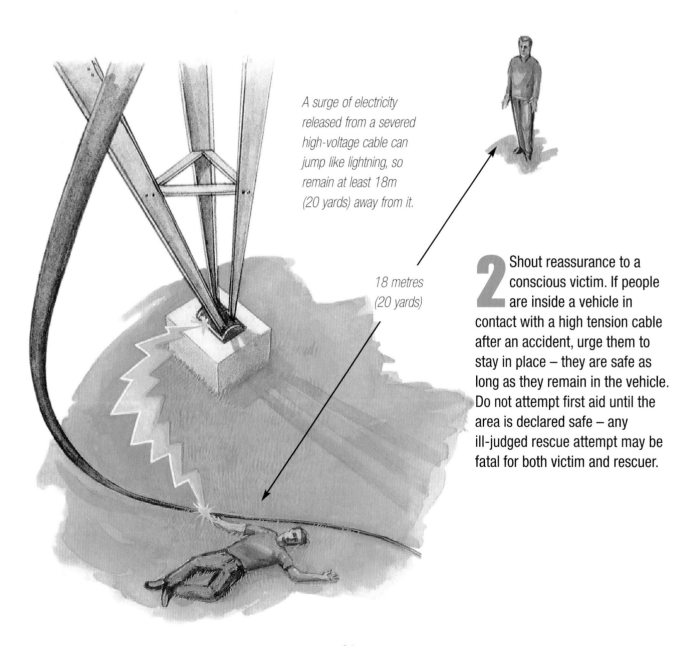

A surge of electricity released from a severed high-voltage cable can jump like lightning, so remain at least 18m (20 yards) away from it.

18 metres (20 yards)

2 Shout reassurance to a conscious victim. If people are inside a vehicle in contact with a high tension cable after an accident, urge them to stay in place – they are safe as long as they remain in the vehicle. Do not attempt first aid until the area is declared safe – any ill-judged rescue attempt may be fatal for both victim and rescuer.

Eye injury

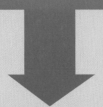

Take action if any of the following occurs:

- Intense pain
- A wound or foreign body in or near to the eye
- The eye appears bloodshot
- Inability to open the affected eye
- Blood or fluid leaking from the eyeball
- Impaired vision
- Itching and watering of the eye

What to look for:

- Spasm of the eyelid, which makes it difficult to open the eye or assess the injury
- Redness of the affected eye with copious watering
- Swelling around the eye

Any eye injury is potentially serious. Direct blows, chemical splashes, intense heat and foreign bodies may all cause complications, including scarring, infection and reduced vision. Ensure the victim receives rapid medical attention.

Chemicals

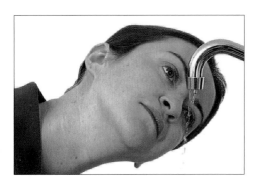

1 Flush the eye under cold running water for ten minutes. Wash from the nose outwards and ensure that water goes under the eyelid. Keep the injured eye low to avoid the water flow contaminating the uninjured eye.

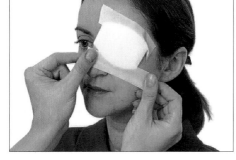

2 If the eye is closed in spasm, hold it open to ensure flushing. Apply a sterile eye pad or dressing secured with lightweight adhesive tape. Take or send a sample of the chemical to hospital with the victim.

Foreign body

1 Tell the victim not to rub the eye. With the victim facing the light, stand behind and gently separate the eyelids. If you see a foreign body on the white of the eye, flush it out with water or lift it off with the corner of a damp handkerchief or tissue.

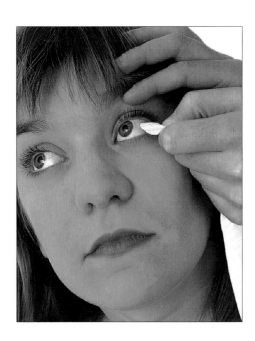

2 If the object is on the coloured part of the eye or is firmly stuck or embedded in the eye, DO NOT attempt to remove it. Cover the eye with a sterile pad secured by adhesive tape and seek urgent medical help.

Facial Injury

Take action if any of the following occurs:

- Pain in the injured area
- An inability to speak, chew or swallow

What to look for:

- Swelling and deformity of the injured area
- Bleeding inside the mouth
- Missing or loose teeth
- Dribbling, if the jaw is fractured

➕ **CALL FOR AN AMBULANCE AT ONCE IF THERE IS CLEAR, STRAW-COLOURED FLUID LEAKING FROM THE EARS OR NOSE – THE VICTIM MAY HAVE A SKULL FRACTURE (SEE PAGE 68).**

Injuries to the face should always be medically assessed to reduce the risks of serious complications or permanent disability. If the nose or mouth is involved, the airway may be obstructed by bleeding. Blindness or a serious head injury can arise from a blow to the cheek or forehead. Injuries that result in loss of consciousness can cause obstruction of the airway by the tongue and inhalation of blood or saliva.

1 If the victim is unconscious, check pulse and breathing and be prepared to start cardiopulmonary resuscitation (see page 13). If there is an injury to the mouth or jaw, ensure that the airway is kept open (see page 8). Place an unconscious victim into the recovery position (see page 11).

2 Help a conscious victim into the most comfortable position – generally sitting with the head forwards. Stop any bleeding with a pad over the wound and apply a cold compress if there is any swelling. Gently support the injured area and arrange immediate transport to hospital.

➕ **IF THE INJURIES INVOLVE THE EYES OR EYE SOCKETS, THE CHEEKBONE, MOUTH, NOSE OR JAW, CALL AN AMBULANCE AS SOON AS POSSIBLE.**

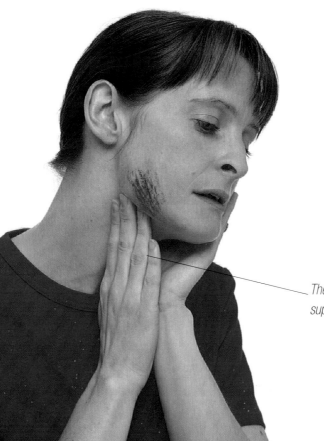

The victim should gently support the injured area.

Fainting

Take action if any of the following occurs:

- Feeling dizzy, faint or lightheaded
- Nausea
- Collapse

What to look for:

- Pale, moist skin
- Restlessness and anxiety
- Slow, sighing breaths
- A very slow pulse

Fainting is common. It can occur if there is a temporary loss of normal blood supply to the brain. Once the victim is lying down, the blood returns to the brain and the person regains consciousness.

1 Try to anticipate the faint and catch the victim, easing him or her to the ground and protecting the head. Raise the legs to restore the circulation. Loosen any tight clothing at neck and waist and ensure there is plenty of fresh air. Stay with the victim until he or she recovers, then give small sips of cool water.

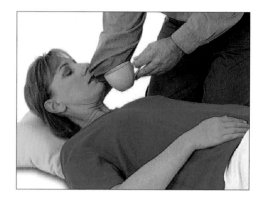

2 When the person feels ready to get up, allow him or her a few minutes to adjust to the change of position. If the victim fails to respond to the spoken voice or touch at any time, move him or her promptly into the recovery position to ensure a clear airway (see page 11).

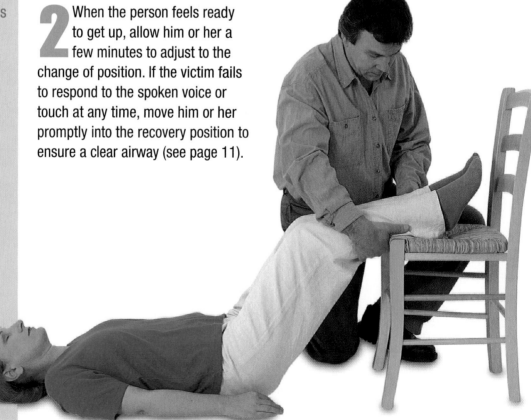

Fits

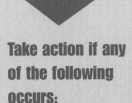

Take action if any of the following occurs:

- Meaningless sounds being made by the victim
- Loss of coordination with staggering and poor balance
- Restlessness and confusion
- Loss of consciousness with a fall to the floor
- Twitching and jerking of some or all limbs with the head tossing from side to side
- Clenching of the teeth with foaming saliva visible
- Loss of bladder and bowel control

Epilepsy is a brain condition in which the victim may have fits. Flashing lights, video games or loud noise can trigger a fit. Some fits follow head injury, poisoning or, in infants, a high temperature (see page 51). In some forms of fits there is no collapse, just a brief disturbance of consciousness, as if the brain has temporarily 'switched off'.

1 Make the area safe to avoid injury while the victim is moving violently on the floor. Move furniture away; place clothing or blankets against heavy items. DO NOT attempt to restrain or move the victim during the fit.

2 When the jerking movements stop, quickly roll the victim onto his or her side and check that the airway is clear (see page 8). The victim is likely to fall asleep at this stage so allow him or her to lie quietly in this position until fully recovered.

✚ **CALL AN AMBULANCE: IF THE VICTIM:**

● **HAS SUSTAINED INJURIES DURING THE FIT;**

● **IS HAVING A FIRST FIT;**

● **IS UNCONSCIOUS FOR MORE THAN TEN MINUTES;**

● **HAS A FURTHER FIT.**

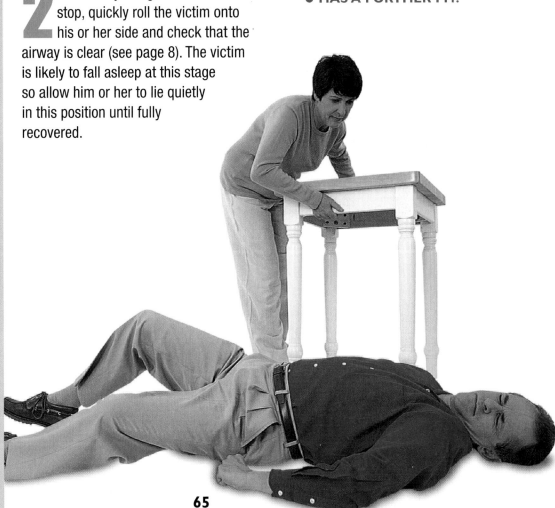

Gas and smoke inhalation

Take action if any of the following occurs:

- Breathing difficulty or breathing failure
- Confusion, listlessness, or 'drunken' behaviour
- Abnormal colour, including pale, blueish or cherry-pink skin
- Burns or soot around the mouth and nose

Carbon monoxide from exhaust fumes or faulty heating appliances is the gas most likely to be inhaled accidentally. This can lead to serious illness, or even death. In most cases, victims of a fire will have inhaled smoke, which may include poisonous fumes given off by burning synthetic fabrics and wall coverings.

1 Do not put yourself in danger. Unless there is a fire, ventilate an enclosed space by opening any doors and windows before entering. If the victim is conscious, help him or her out of the contaminated area into fresh air.

✚ **SEND SOMEONE TO CALL AN AMBULANCE AS SOON AS POSSIBLE. MEDICAL ASSESSMENT IS VITAL, BECAUSE SERIOUS COMPLICATIONS CAN RESULT FROM THE INHALATION OF A TOXIC SUBSTANCE.**

✚ **DO NOT ENTER A CONFINED SPACE FILLED WITH GAS OR SMOKE WITHOUT PROPER SAFETY EQUIPMENT – AWAIT ARRIVAL OF EMERGENCY SERVICES.**

2 Lift or drag an unconscious victim into the fresh air. Check the airway (see page 8) and begin CPR (cardiopulmonary resuscitation, see page 13) if necessary. Once breathing is regular, place the victim in the recovery position (see page 11).

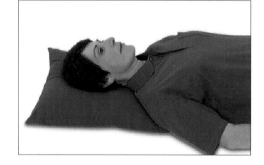

3 If the victim is conscious, monitor pulse and breathing until the ambulance arrives. Treat any other injuries such as burns.

Gunshot wounds

Take action if any
of the following
occurs:

- Pain
- Faintness
- Nausea
- Collapse

What to look for:

- Bleeding
- Entry and exit wounds
- Pale, cold and clammy skin
- Rapid breathing and a rapid, weak pulse

Bullet wounds can cause serious internal injuries and infection. Often there is only a small wound at the entry point, but a large exit wound with extensive tissue damage. If the bullet lodges inside the body, there may be only a small entry wound, but massive internal damage is likely.

✚ **CALL AN AMBULANCE IMMEDIATELY.**

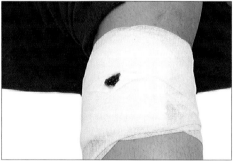

1 Check the victim's response to simple instructions. If the victim fails to respond promptly, check the airway (see page 8) and give CPR (cardiopulmonary resuscitation, see page 13) if needed. Place an unconscious victim in the recovery position.

Help a conscious victim into a comfortable position.

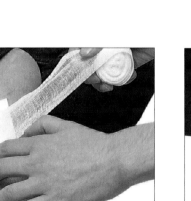

2 Check for entry and exit wounds and apply firm pressure to control any bleeding: if the wound is open and deep, use several large, sterile, bulky pads.

3 If there is a broken bone with the wound, avoid moving the injured part. Apply pressure on either side of the wound and build up padding around it. Hold the padding in position with a bandage that is applied in a criss-cross formation (see page 35).

Head injury

Take action if any of the following occurs:

- Headache
- Nausea or vomiting
- Blurred or double vision
- Numbness, tingling or loss of power in the limbs
- Alterations in consciousness

What to look for:

- Total or partial loss of consciousness
- Loss of short-term memory
- Loss of hand-to-eye coordination
- Signs of weakness or paralysis down one side
- Unequal size of the pupils
- Noisy breathing, flushed face and a strong, slow pulse

Any head injury is potentially serious and some are life-threatening. Seek prompt medical care to avoid permanent disability. While waiting for an ambulance to arrive, observe the victim closely. This is essential to give early warning of any complications that might lead to permanent brain damage.

✚ **CALL FOR AN AMBULANCE AS SOON AS POSSIBLE. STAY WITH THE VICTIM UNTIL IT ARRIVES.**

1 Check the victim's response to simple instructions such as, 'Squeeze my hand. Now let it go.' If the victim fails to respond promptly, check the airway and quickly place him or her into the recovery position (see page 11). Be prepared to give CPR (cardiopulmonary resuscitation, see page 13) if necessary.

2 If a victim who has been unconscious wakes up within a few minutes, maintain very close observation in case they lose consciousness again.

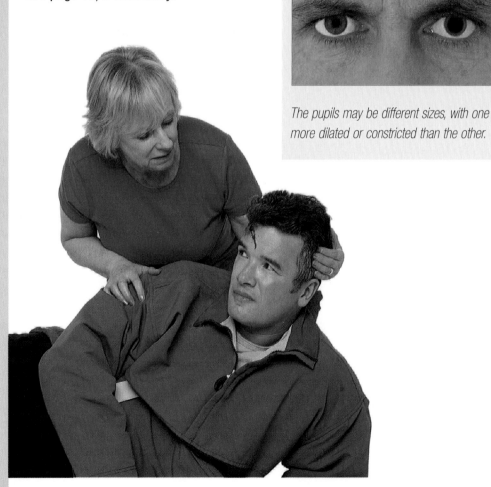

The pupils may be different sizes, with one more dilated or constricted than the other.

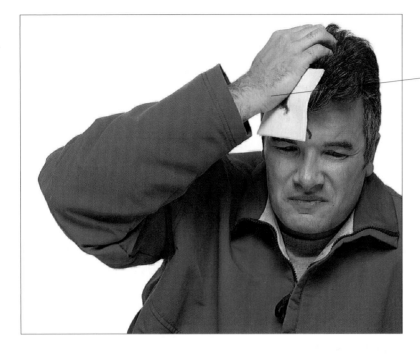

Ask the victim to hold the dressing in place.

➕ **ALL HEAD INJURIES, EVEN THOSE THAT APPEAR TO BE MINOR WITH NO ABNORMAL SYMPTOMS OR SIGNS, SHOULD BE CHECKED BY A DOCTOR BECAUSE OF THE RISK OF COMPLICATIONS.**

➕ **NOTE DOWN YOUR OBSERVATIONS OF THE VICTIM SINCE THE INCIDENT AND PASS THEM ONTO THE AMBULANCE CREW WHEN THEY ARRIVE.**

3 Help a conscious victim into a comfortable position and keep a close watch while treating any superficial injuries. Check for any warning signs of serious injury, including loss of short-term memory and hand-to-eye coordination.

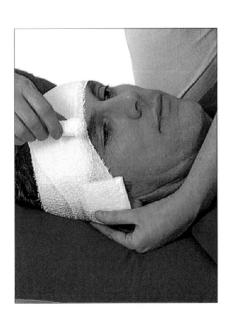

4 Check for head wounds. Control any bleeding by covering the wound with a sterile dressing and applying pressure with the palm of your hand. If any fluid is draining from one ear, apply a sterile pad secured with a roller bandage (see page 27). Do not pack the ear canal. Ask the victim to tilt the head towards the injured side.

5 Check the victim at frequent intervals and note any changes in his or her conscious state and coordination.

Heart attack

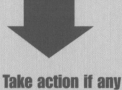

Take action if any of the following occurs:

- Severe chest pain: this may be tight, crushing or vice-like; it may occur in the centre of the chest or around the chest; it may go up the jaw and down one arm (especially the left)
- Breathlessness
- Nausea
- Sudden giddiness or faintness

What to look for:

- Pale, greyish skin with a cold and clammy feel
- Rapid, weak pulse
- Shivering and anxiety
- Collapse

A heart attack is often due to a blood clot causing a blockage in one of the coronary arteries which supplies blood to the heart muscle. If urgent medical treatment is obtained, the victim may make a full recovery.

1 Help the victim into a position of rest, preferably sitting or half-reclining with the head and shoulders supported.

✚ **CALL AN AMBULANCE AT ONCE AND STATE THAT THE VICTIM MAY HAVE HAD A HEART ATTACK.**

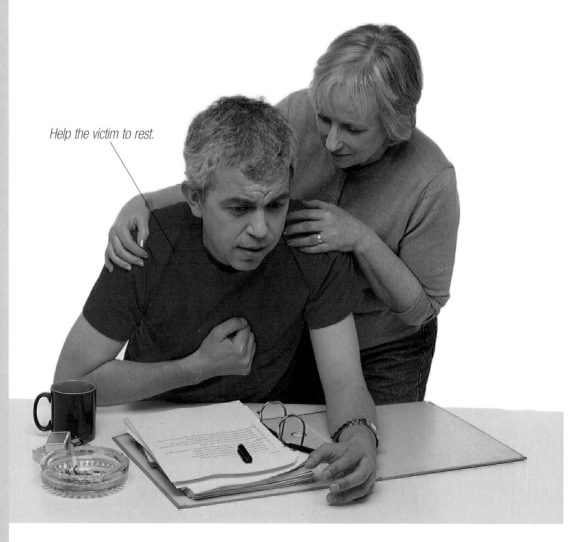

Help the victim to rest.

2 If collapse occurs, check that the airway is clear and open (see page 8). Be ready to give CPR (cardiopulmonary resuscitation, see page 13) if needed. Place the victim in the recovery position (see page 11).

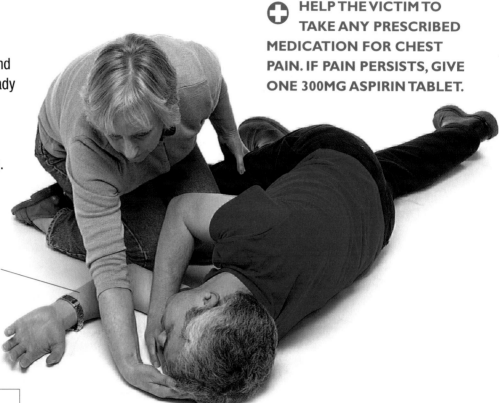

✚ HELP THE VICTIM TO TAKE ANY PRESCRIBED MEDICATION FOR CHEST PAIN. IF PAIN PERSISTS, GIVE ONE 300MG ASPIRIN TABLET.

Quickly place an unconscious victim in the recovery position.

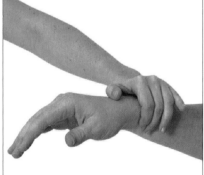

3 Keep monitoring the pulse and respiration until the ambulance arrives. If possible, make a note of these observations and send this to the hospital with the victim.

Heart attack risk factors

High blood pressure
This causes hardening of the arteries. Adults should have regular check-ups.

Smoking
Nicotine narrows blood vessels and can raise blood pressure, forcing the heart to work harder.

High blood cholesterol
Eating saturated fat like butter and lard, clogs up the arteries. Unsaturated fats such as sunflower and olive oil are better.

Obesity
Weight control through a healthy diet is important because obesity increases the workload on the heart and causes high blood pressure.

Lack of exercise
Healthy hearts need oxygen. Regular aerobic exercise, such as cycling, swimming or walking, will improve the efficiency of the heart and lungs. Exercise for 30 minutes at least three times a week.

Heat exhaustion

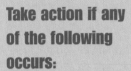

Take action if any of the following occurs:

- Exhaustion and thirst
- Headache, nausea and dizzy spells
- Cramps

What to look for:

- Profuse sweating
- Cool, moist and pale skin
- A rapid and weak pulse
- Confusion

Heat exhaustion is the most common form of heat-related illness. It develops gradually as the body's heat-regulating mechanism is overloaded, resulting in excessive fluid and salt loss from the body through perspiration.

1 Call for an ambulance as soon as possible. Then help the victim to lie down in a shaded place. Loosen any tight clothing at neck and waist and raise both legs.

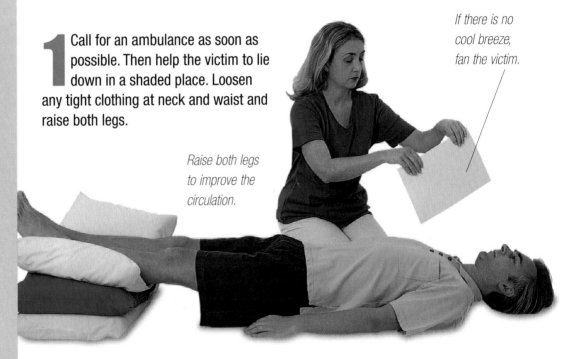

If there is no cool breeze, fan the victim.

Raise both legs to improve the circulation.

2 If the victim is conscious, give him or her plenty of liquid to drink. Give water, sweet fluids or a weak salt solution of one teaspoon of salt dissolved in one litre (1¾pts) of water.

✚ **SEEK URGENT MEDICAL ADVICE TO AVOID THE ONSET OF HEAT STROKE. NOTE ANY CHANGE IN THE VICTIM'S CONDITION AND RECORD ANY SIGNS OF DETERIORATION.**

3 If the victim becomes unconscious, check the airway is clear and open (see page 8) and be prepared to resuscitate if necessary (see page 10). Place the victim in the recovery position (see page 11).

Heat stroke

Take action if any of the following occurs:

- Headache and dizzy spells
- Feeling hot and very dry

What to look for:

- A high temperature with a red, hot and dry skin
- Restlessness and confusion
- A strong, bounding pulse
- Deteriorating level of response

Heat stroke is due to failure of the body's temperature control, resulting in dangerous overheating. Sweating – the body's natural cooling system – ceases, and the body temperature may rise to 40°C (104°F) or more. Heat stroke develops rapidly and requires prompt treatment by rapid cooling.

✚ **CALL AN AMBULANCE IMMEDIATELY.**

1 Move the victim to a cool place. Remove as much outer clothing as possible.

Help to cool the body by removing the victim's outer clothing.

2 If the victim is fully conscious, give frequent sips of cool water. Wrap the victim in a cold, wet sheet or towel, and keep it wet until the temperature falls to 38°C (100°F). The wet cloth can then be replaced with a dry one. Monitor until help arrives, and be prepared to restart active cooling if the person's temperature rises again.

3 If the victim becomes unconscious, check that the airway is clear (see page 8). Be ready to start CPR (cardiopulmonary resuscitation, see page 13) immediately. Place the victim in the recovery position (see page 11).

If the victim's temperature is over 38°C (100°F), cover him or her with a wet sheet, and fan.

Hip and pelvis injury

Take action if any of the following occurs:

- Severe pain at the site of injury
- Inability to walk
- Nausea, giddiness or faintness

What to look for:

- An injured leg with the knee and foot turned outwards
- Paleness, with cold and clammy skin
- A swollen and bruised hip joint

Hip injuries occur most commonly in elderly people after a fall, particularly in women with osteoporosis. The area around the hip will be tender and swollen with blood which has leaked from damaged blood vessels. The victim needs very gentle handling with the minimum of movement to avoid further blood loss and the risk of severe shock.

1 Reassure the victim that he or she will not be moved until an ambulance arrives. Try to provide some support for the injured limb by placing a folded blanket or rolled-up clothing gently alongside the leg. Do NOT raise the leg.

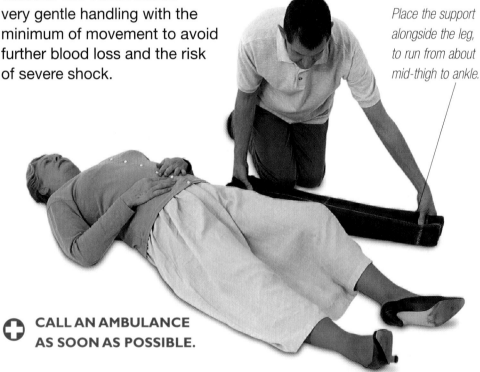

Place the support alongside the leg, to run from about mid-thigh to ankle.

✚ **CALL AN AMBULANCE AS SOON AS POSSIBLE.**

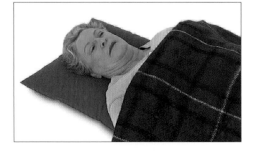

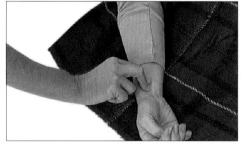

2 Cover the victim lightly with a blanket to reduce heat loss. If lying on a cold or wet surface, gently slide a blanket or cloth under the head, body and uninjured leg, but DO NOT move the injured limb.

3 Stay with the victim until an ambulance arrives. Check the pulse rate at intervals and watch for signs of shock (see page 85). Do not give the victim any food or drink in case an anaesthetic is needed.

74

Hyperventilation

Take action if any of the following occurs:

- A choking feeling or an inability to breathe properly
- Tightness in the chest
- Extreme fear and apprehension
- Tingling and spasm in the toes and fingers
- Dizziness, trembling or cramps

What to look for:

- Unnaturally fast breathing
- Clawlike finger spasms or shaking
- Screaming, shouting or crying

Hyperventilation or overbreathing is usually due to fear, anxiety or panic. Breathing becomes extremely rapid and the person undergoes a temporary loss of control as a result of an over-reaction to a stressful or emotional situation. The overbreathing causes a temporary imbalance of oxygen and carbon dioxide in the body. Although the situation may appear to be serious, recovery is usually rapid once breathing stabilizes. Symptoms are often dramatic but the victim is fully aware throughout the attack. It is important to remember that some serious medical conditions can cause similar rapid and shallow breathing. If symptoms persist, seek medical attention.

1 Stay calm and speak kindly but firmly. Remove the victim from any source of distress, and keep onlookers away. Reassure the victim that the symptoms will disappear once breathing returns to normal.

2 Encourage the victim to breathe more slowly by counting and deliberately setting a slower rate, telling the victim to breathe on your count. Continue this until breathing is slow and regular.

➕ **DO NOT TRY TO RESTRAIN THE VICTIM. DO NOT SLAP THE VICTIM'S FACE OR THROW WATER OVER HIM OR HER.**

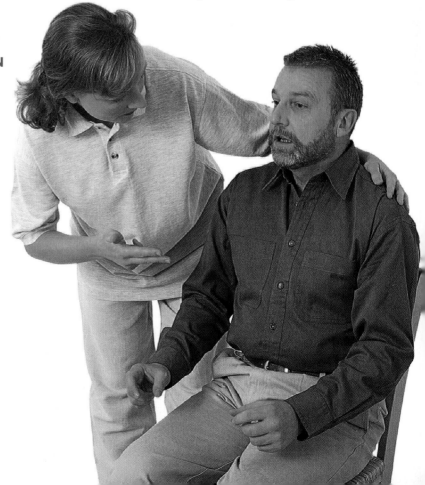

Hypothermia

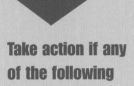

Take action if any of the following occurs:

- Feeling very cold and shivery
- Numbness of the face, fingers and toes
- Apathy or confusion
- Lethargy

What to look for:

- Cold, dry skin
- Mental confusion
- Failing consciousness
- Slow, shallow breathing
- A slow pulse that becomes irregular

Hypothermia is a medical emergency that occurs when the body cannot produce enough heat to stay warm. If a victim of severe hypothermia is not given prompt first aid and medical care, the heart may cease to function normally and death can occur.

A sleeping bag is ideal for raising the body temperature.

Give sips of warm liquid.

1 If indoors, an elderly victim should only be rewarmed gradually, using layers of blankets, as a sudden change in temperature can be dangerous. Give sips of warm (not hot) liquid, and high-energy foods such as chocolate. Put the victim to bed until help arrives.

2 If the victim is out in the open, find or improvise some shelter. If possible remove any wet clothing and cover the victim with dry clothes or blankets. If not, use extra clothing or blankets. Cover the victim's head and place fabric or newspapers underneath to insulate from cold ground. Lie beside the victim and use your own body heat to transfer warmth.

3 Move an unconscious victim into the recovery position (see page 11) and be prepared to start CPR (cardiopulmonary resuscitation, see page 13), if necessary.

✚ **CALL AN AMBULANCE AS SOON AS POSSIBLE.**

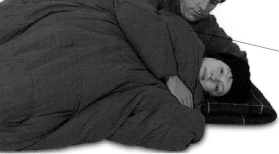

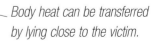

Body heat can be transferred by lying close to the victim.

Hysteria

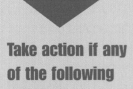

Take action if any of the following occurs:

- Extreme fear and apprehension
- A choking feeling or an inability to breathe properly
- Tingling and spasm in the fingers
- Dizziness or an inability to move

What to look for:

- Screaming, shouting and crying
- Rapid and shallow breathing
- Clawlike finger spasms

Hysteria results from an over-reaction to a stressful or emotional situation. It can be seen as a temporary loss of control; symptoms are often more dramatic if there are any bystanders. Although the situation may appear to be serious, the victim rarely suffers any harm and will remain aware of any hazards throughout the attack.

IF THE VICTIM CANNOT BE CALMED OR IS HAVING BREATHING DIFFICULTY OR SEVERE FINGER SPASMS, CALL AN AMBULANCE.

1 Isolate the victim from any bystanders and give him or her calm and positive reassurance. Stay with the victim and observe any behaviour changes until the attack subsides.

2 Try to help the victim by counting out loud together to slow down his or her breathing rate. DO NOT use a paper bag for rebreathing – this causes serious complications in some people.

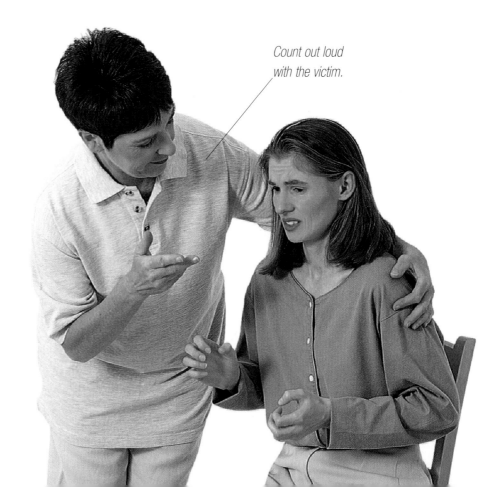

Count out loud with the victim.

Leg and knee injury

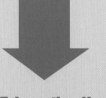

Take action if any of the following occurs:

- A recent blow or twisting injury to the knee or leg
- Pain in and around the joint or injury site
- 'Locking' of the knee joint, or pain on trying to move or straighten the leg
- Swelling of the knee
- Loss of power and function in the affected limb
- Nausea, vomiting or dizziness

What to look for:
- Swelling
- Deformity of the knee or limb
- Pale, cold and clammy skin
- An injured leg turned or rolled outwards
- Shortening of the injured limb due to muscle spasm

Knees can be injured in many ways – road accidents, sports activities or a heavy fall at home or work. In such accidents the kneecap is often injured, and occasionally the hinge joint beneath is hurt as well.

KNEE INJURY

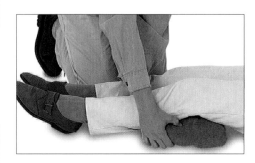

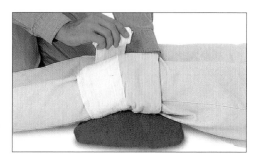

1 Help the victim to lie down, steadying and supporting the injured limb. DO NOT attempt to straighten or bend the knee. Place padding or rolled-up clothing under the joint for support.

2 Hold the padding in place with a roller bandage (see page 25). Do not give the victim any food or drink in case an anaesthetic is needed to treat the injury. Call an ambulance or arrange transport to hospital.

LEG INJURY

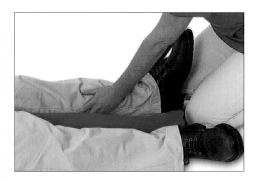

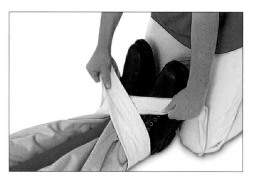

1 Help the victim to lie down while supporting the injured limb. If it is positioned at an awkward angle, gently place the leg in the direction of the foot – stop if this causes pain. Place padding along the inside of the injured leg. Position the other leg alongside.

2 Slide bandages above and below the knees to splint the legs together, then bandage the ankles together using a criss-cross pattern. Maintain a firm pull until the knot is secure. If this adds to the pain, stop at once and support the limb as it lies.

Muscle injury

Take action if any of the following occurs:

- Pain at the injury site
- Pressure beneath the skin
- Reduced function of the injured part

What to look for

- Swelling of the injured area
- Tissues that feel hard to the touch
- Blueish discoloration around the injury site

There are many muscles, tendons and ligaments in the leg, and these are easily damaged. Deep bleeding can fill the tissue spaces with blood and may be felt as a hard or corklike sensation.

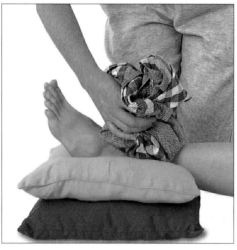

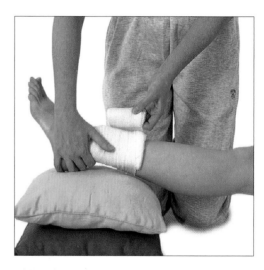

1 If the injury has only just occurred, first stop any further bleeding into the tissues by raising the limb on cushions or rolled-up clothing and applying an ice pack or cold compress (see page 31).

2 Apply firm pressure to the injured area with padding or bandages. This will help to reduce pain and swelling and to lessen later bruising. Advise the victim to rest the part and to seek medical attention.

✚ AFTER FIRST AID TREATMENT, SEEK MEDICAL ADVICE TO AVOID LONG-TERM DISABILITY AND COMPLICATIONS.

Nosebleed and injury

Take action if any of the following occurs:

- Bleeding from the nose
- Blood trickling down the back of the throat
- Pain
- Difficulty breathing through the nose

What to look for:

- Obvious deformity of the nose
- Bleeding or clear nasal discharge
- Swelling or bruising

✚ **IF BLEEDING HAS NOT STOPPED AFTER 30 MINUTES, SEEK MEDICAL ADVICE.**

There are many small blood vessels close to the surface in the nose which may be damaged by an impact or by sneezing, picking or blowing the nose. Nosebleeds are rarely serious. However, if the skull is fractured after a head injury (see page 68), a bloodstained watery fluid may drain from the nose and be mistaken for a nosebleed. If this is a possibility, seek urgent medical advice.

NOSEBLEED

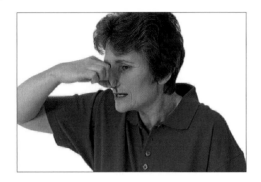

1 Sit the victim down with the head tilted forwards. Ask him or her to pinch both nostrils together and breathe through the mouth. Do not plug the nose with a dressing or cotton wool.

2 Keep the nostrils pinched for at least ten minutes to allow a firm clot to form. If bleeding continues when the pressure is removed, reapply the pressure for a further ten minutes. If bleeding still continues, seek urgent medical attention.

3 When the bleeding has stopped, give the victim a moist tissue to clean around the nose but not inside the nostrils. To avoid repeat nosebleeds, advise the victim not to take strenuous exercise and not to blow the nose for several hours.

FRACTURED NOSE

1 Immediately apply a cold compress (see page 31) to the bridge of the nose to reduce swelling. If necessary, treat any nosebleed.

2 Arrange for the victim to go to hospital for medical attention as soon as possible. Do not give the person any food or drink in case an anaesthetic is necessary.

✚ **IF THERE IS CLEAR OR STRAW-COLOURED FLUID DRAINING FROM THE NOSE, CALL AN AMBULANCE AT ONCE.**

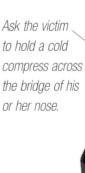

Ask the victim to hold a cold compress across the bridge of his or her nose.

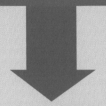

Overdose

A drug overdose may be deliberate or accidental, and may involve prescription drugs, over-the-counter medicines, illegal street drugs or inhaled solvents such as glue or lighter fuel. The signs vary considerably, depending on what type of drug has been taken.

Take action if any of the following occurs:

- Slurred speech
- Staggering or loss of coordination
- Dilation or constriction of the pupils of the eyes
- Vomiting
- Confusion or delirium
- Hallucinations
- Slow, shallow breathing
- Total or partial loss of consciousness

➕ CALL FOR AN AMBULANCE AS SOON AS POSSIBLE.

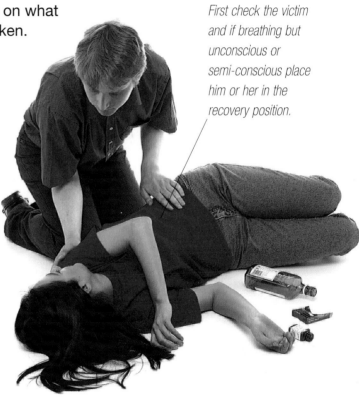

First check the victim and if breathing but unconscious or semi-conscious place him or her in the recovery position.

1 If the victim is unconscious or semi-conscious, check the airway (see page 8) and be prepared to start resuscitation (see page 10). Place the victim into the recovery position (see page 11).

2 If the victim is conscious, be prepared for angry or violent behaviour. Try to persuade the victim to go to hospital. Be ready to start resuscitation if there is a sudden deterioration in the victim's condition.

➕ DO NOT LEAVE THE VICTIM UNTIL THE AMBULANCE ARRIVES.

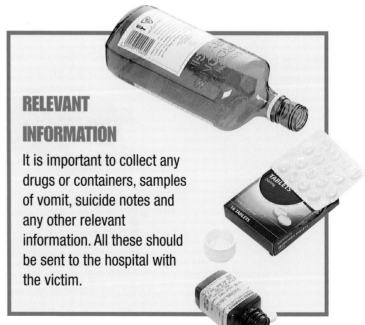

RELEVANT INFORMATION

It is important to collect any drugs or containers, samples of vomit, suicide notes and any other relevant information. All these should be sent to the hospital with the victim.

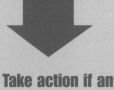

Take action if any of the following occurs:

Poison absorbed

- An irritating rash at the contact site
- Moderate to severe pain at contact site
- Nausea, headache or dizziness

Poison inhaled

- Breathing difficulty or breathing failure
- Listlessness, confusion or 'drunken' behaviour
- Abnormal colour, including pale, cherry-pink or blueish skin

What to look for:

- Area of redness, blisters or a rash
- Distress

ABSORBED POISONS

Some substances found around the home can be highly toxic if absorbed through the skin. These include insecticides and weedkillers. Household chemicals can also cause severe contact burns (see page 41).

⊕ **SEND SOMEONE TO CALL AN AMBULANCE AS SOON AS POSSIBLE.**

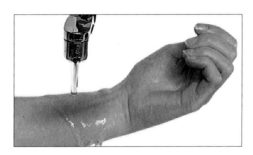

Ask the victim to remove all contaminated clothing immediately. Wash affected areas of skin thoroughly under running water.

Emergency procedures

If a victim becomes unconscious after absorbing or inhaling poison, check the airway (see page 8) and be ready to begin CPR (cardiopulmonary resuscitation, see page 13). Place in the recovery position (see page 11) until help arrives.

INHALED POISONS

There are many substances around the home from which poisonous fumes can be inhaled accidentally. In a fire, smoke from burning plastics and synthetic furnishings is likely to contain toxic vapours. Carbon monoxide from faulty heating appliances can also cause severe poisoning.

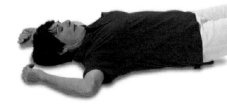

1 If the victim is conscious, help them out of the contaminated area into fresh air. Drag an unconscious victim away by the feet or shoulders. Keep the victim under close observation outside until the ambulance arrives.

Poison swallowed

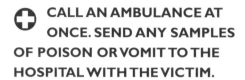

Take action if any of the following occurs:

- Nausea
- Abdominal cramps

What to look for:

- Vomiting
- Seizures or convulsions
- Burns around the mouth and nose
- Diarrhoea
- Drowsiness or loss of consciousness
- Confusion or hallucinations
- A used container; berries

Poison is most often taken by mouth, especially by young children. If a poison has been swallowed, do not give any food or fluid unless directed to do so, as this can cause complications.

1 If the victim is conscious, ask what type of poison has been taken, how much and how long ago.

✚ **DO NOT TRY TO INDUCE VOMITING.**

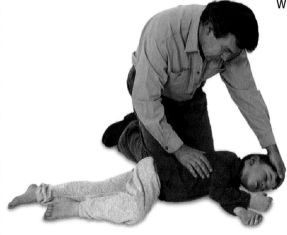

✚ **CALL AN AMBULANCE AT ONCE. SEND ANY SAMPLES OF POISON OR VOMIT TO THE HOSPITAL WITH THE VICTIM.**

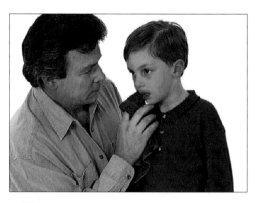

2 If there is any redness or signs of burning around the mouth or on the lips, wash the area well with plenty of cold water.

3 If the victim is unconscious, check the airway (see page 8). If necessary, begin CPR (cardiopulmonary resuscitation, see page 13) promptly. Avoid contamination by using a plastic face shield, if available. Place the victim in the recovery position (see page 11) until medical help arrives.

AVOIDING ACCIDENTS

- Keep dangerous substances out of sight and out of reach of children.
- Keep all medications in a locked medicine cabinet.
- Chemicals should be left in their original, correctly labelled containers and should never be mixed or transferred into food or soft drink containers that might be attractive to a child.
- Never mix cleaning products together. Store them in a locked cupboard or on a shelf that is inaccessible to children.
- Keep all medicines and household substances in childproof containers.
- Return out-of-date medicines or those no longer needed to a pharmacy so that they can be disposed of safely.

Severed limb

Take action if any
of the following
occurs:

- A limb or body part is severed
- Bleeding
- Shock

✚ **CALL AN AMBULANCE IMMEDIATELY. REMEMBER TO MENTION THAT AN AMPUTATION IS INVOLVED.**

If a limb or digit is severed in an injury, there is a chance that surgery can rejoin the amputated part. However, for this to be successful, immediate care of both the stump and severed part is essential. Controlling the bleeding is the first priority in any emergency care.

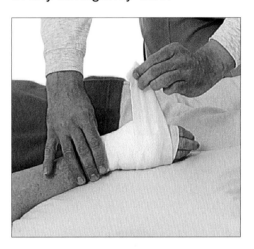

Blow into the plastic bag before tying, to create an air cushion for the severed part.

✚ **SEND THE SEVERED PART TO HOSPITAL WITH THE VICTIM.**

1 Lie the victim down and control bleeding by placing a clean pad over the stump and applying pressure. Do not use a tourniquet. Raise the injured part. When bleeding slows, secure the pad with a bandage, or apply a sterile dressing.

2 Rescue the severed part – in this case, a thumb. Place it in a plastic bag tied to retain an air cushion around the part. Alternatively, wrap the part in cling film surrounded by gauze or soft fabric. Place the wrapped part in a container filled with crushed ice, or cold water with added ice cubes. Do not allow ice to come into direct contact with the severed part.

3 Treat for shock if necessary. Reassure the victim until the ambulance arrives. If possible, label the container holding the severed part with the victim's name and the time of injury.

4 Check the victim's pulse rate every ten minutes and note any changes to report to the ambulance staff. Do not give the victim any food or drink in case it is necessary to give him or her an anaesthetic.

Shock

Take action if any of the following occurs:

- Feeling weak, faint and giddy
- Nausea and even vomiting
- Pain (depending on the problem)

What to look for:

- Pale, cold and clammy skin
- Rapid and shallow breathing
- Yawning or sighing ('air hunger')
- Weak, rapid pulse

Shock happens when the body's circulation system fails, endangering the blood supply to vital organs such as the heart and brain. It can occur after severe injury or illness, including heart attack, infection, allergy or blood loss. It is not the same as psychological shock. Without treatment the blood supply can weaken until the victim falls unconscious and may die.

1 Treat any obvious cause of shock, such as heavy bleeding. Lie the victim down on a blanket (to protect from the cold ground). Raise the legs high and keep the head low. Loosen any tight clothing at neck, chest and waist.

2 Keep the victim warm by covering with coats or blankets. Do not use direct heat, such as hot-water bottles.

3 Keep checking pulse, breathing and level of response. Be prepared to resuscitate if necessary (see page 10). Turn an unconscious victim into the recovery position (see page 11).

➕ **CALL FOR AN AMBULANCE AS SOON AS POSSIBLE. AVOID GIVING ANY FOOD OR DRINK IN CASE AN ANAESTHETIC IS NEEDED TO TREAT THE UNDERLYING CONDITION.**

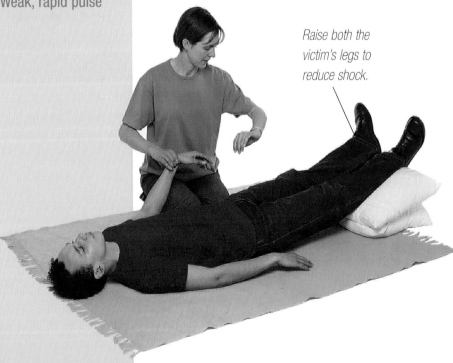

Raise both the victim's legs to reduce shock.

Sprains and strains

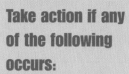

Take action if any of the following occurs:

Sprains

- Sudden pain in and around a joint
- Nausea, giddiness or fainting
- Pain increased by movement or weight bearing
- Loss of power and function in the joint

Strains

- Sudden, sharp pain in the area
- Stiffness and swelling
- Cramp in the injured tissue

What to look for:

Sprains

- Swelling, with some bruising later

Strains

- Cramping spasm of the injured area

SPRAINS

A sprain occurs when a ligament – a tough band of fibrous tissue connecting bones at a joint – is suddenly overstretched. Provided the ligament has not been torn, gradual healing will occur. The most common places for a sprain are the ankle and wrist. However, as some sprains are associated with other injuries, it can be difficult to tell one from a fracture (broken bone). If in doubt, always seek medical advice.

1 Help the victim into the most comfortable position possible. Avoid moving or touching the injured area more than necessary. Help the victim to steady and support the injured part on a pillow or other soft support to rest it. For a back strain, help the victim to lie down on the ground or a firm mattress.

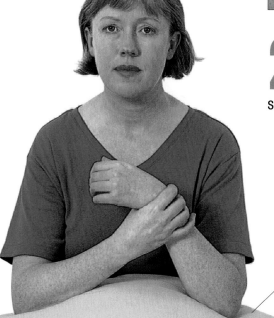

Treatment of sprains and strains involves the **RICE** procedure:

Rest the injured part.
Ice or a cold compress should be applied.
Compress the injury.
Elevate the injured part.

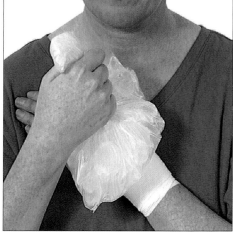

2 Apply an ice pack or cold compress (see page 31) to the injured area to reduce pain, swelling and bruising.

Rest the injured limb on a soft support.

STRAINS

Strains happen when a muscle is stretched or overworked. They usually occur in the neck, lower back, thigh or calf as a result of a sudden jarring movement.

1 If possible, apply gentle pressure to the injured part, using soft padding secured with a bandage. This will also help to control swelling and pain.

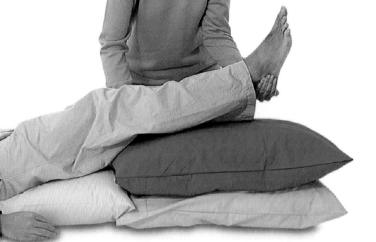

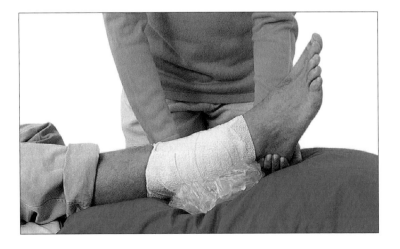

EXCEPT FOR MINOR INJURIES, SEEK MEDICAL ADVICE IN CASE A FRACTURE IS PRESENT.

2 Elevate an injured limb on a soft pillow or cushion to reduce blood flow and help minimize bruising. Place an ice pack around the bandaged area to bring further relief.

3 Advise the victim to rest and to seek medical attention if symptoms do not improve within four to five hours.

Stroke

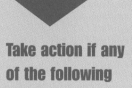

Take action if any of the following occurs:

- Weakness or numbness down one side of the body
- Severe headache
- Confusion – which may seem like drunkenness
- Reducing level of consciousness
- Slurred speech

What to look for:

- Loss of muscle tone in the face muscles
- An inability to speak coherently
- Saliva dribbling from the mouth
- Unequal pupil sizes
- Loss of bladder or bowel control
- Unconsciousness

A stroke occurs when a blood vessel in the brain bursts or is blocked by a blood clot. A part of the brain is then starved of oxygen, resulting in paralysis down one side of the body and loss of the ability to speak. A minor stroke may last for only a few minutes, with the victim making a complete recovery.

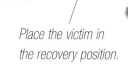

Place the victim in the recovery position.

1 If the victim is unconscious, check that the airway is clear (see page 8). Be ready to give CPR (cardiopulmonary resuscitation, see page 13). Turn the victim into the recovery position (see page 11) once breathing and pulse are established.

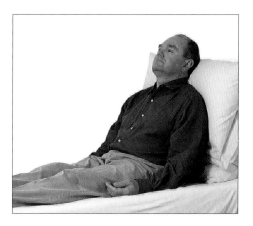

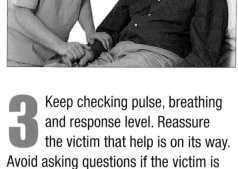

2 Sit or lie a conscious victim with the head and shoulders slightly raised. Loosen any tight clothing and tilt the head slightly to one side. Use a towel to absorb dribbling.

3 Keep checking pulse, breathing and response level. Reassure the victim that help is on its way. Avoid asking questions if the victim is having difficulty speaking.

✚ **CALL AN AMBULANCE AT ONCE – TREATMENT WITHIN TWO HOURS MAY AVOID PERMANENT DISABILITY.**

4 Remember that the victim may still hear and understand you, even if he cannot respond. Do not give any food or drink because swallowing may be impaired.

Suffocation

Take action if any
of the following
occurs:

- Obvious threat to
  air supply
- Noisy or difficult
  breathing
- Blue or grey colour
  of lips and skin
- Unconsciousness

What to look for:

- Discoloration of lips,
  skin or tongue
- Flaring of the
  nostrils
- Drawing in of the
  chest wall between
  the ribs and above
  the collar bones

Suffocation occurs when oxygen is prevented from entering the airways. It may result from a blockage such as choking (see page 46), smothering, a heavy weight crushing the chest or swelling of the throat. It can also occur when there is not enough oxygen in the air breathed in, for example with fumes, or because the body cannot absorb oxygen, as in carbon monoxide poisoning (see page 66).

1 Remove any obvious obstruction to breathing, for example by clearing the airway (see page 8) or moving the victim into fresh air.

2 If the victim is unconscious, open the airway (see page 8). Check for breathing, and start CPR (cardiopulmonary resuscitation, see page 13) if necessary. Once the pulse and breathing are established, place the victim in the recovery position (see page 11).

✚ **CALL AN AMBULANCE IMMEDIATELY IF A VICTIM HAS BEEN UNCONSCIOUS.**

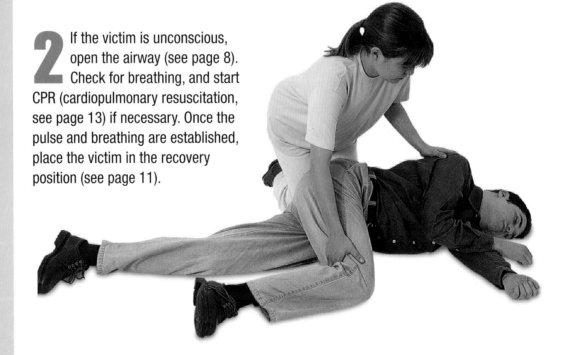

3 If the victim is conscious, check pulse and breathing regularly and call a doctor – even if the victim appears to be fully recovered.

Sunburn

Take action if any of the following occurs:

- Pain
- Heat in the burned area
- Redness or tightness of the skin

What to look for:

- Red and possibly blistered skin
- Skin tender to the touch

Direct exposure to the sun in the middle of the day can cause sunburn after only 20 minutes. Although sunscreen will protect the skin for a short time, it should always be reapplied after swimming. Young children in particular may receive serious and painful burns unless they are closely supervised.

1 Cover the burnt area with loose fabric while helping the victim into a cool or shaded place, preferably indoors. Cool the skin by sponging or soaking in cold water for ten minutes. Help the victim to change into loose clothes, and to rest without putting pressure on the sunburned area. Encourage the person to take frequent sips of cool water.

✚ **WHEN THE VICTIM IS UNDER FIVE YEARS OF AGE, OR IS ELDERLY, SEEK PROMPT MEDICAL ADVICE IF HEADACHE, A RAISED TEMPERATURE OR RESTLESSNESS DEVELOPS.**

2 Apply an after-sun cream, calamine lotion or anaesthetic spray to the painful areas to soothe the skin. If in doubt, seek the advice of a pharmacist.

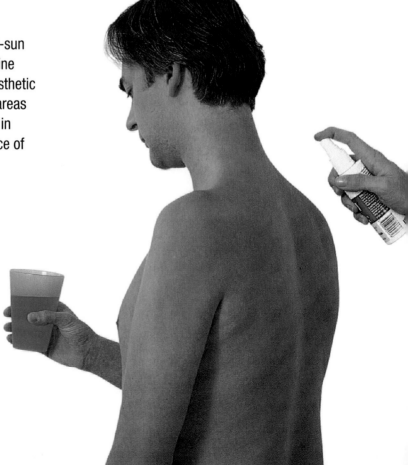

A cool drink will help to rehydrate the victim.

Tooth injury

CONTACT A DENTIST TO ARRANGE FOR AN IMMEDIATE APPOINTMENT.

Take action if any of the following occurs:

- Pain
- Bleeding inside the mouth

What to look for:

- Missing or broken tooth
- Bleeding tooth socket
- Irregularity of other teeth

If an adult tooth is chipped or fractured, prompt dental care can often restore or save it. If a tooth is knocked out of the gum, it may be possible to reimplant it successfully. Do not wash the tooth or try to wipe it clean as this can destroy the membrane around its base. Do not try to replace a child's milk tooth.

1 Help the victim to sit or lie down comfortably with the head tilted forward and towards the injured side. If a tooth has been knocked out, find it and attempt to replace it in the socket as soon as possible.

2 Hold the tooth firmly and carefully position it into the socket. Wrap a gauze pad over the tooth and ask the victim to keep this in place by gripping between upper and lower teeth. Ensure that the victim seeks immediate advice from a dentist or hospital.

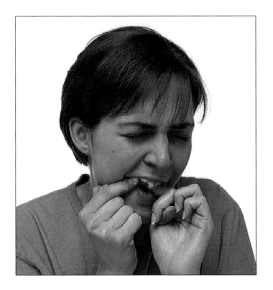

Ask the victim to bite on a pad held over the replaced tooth, to keep it in place.

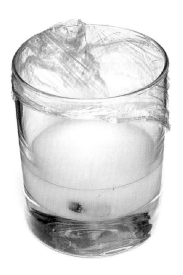

3 If the tooth cannot be replaced because of pain or extensive injury, ask the victim to hold it in the mouth, or place it in milk or water, to keep the roots moist until dental care is available. If there is any bleeding, make a firm pad from a rolled tissue or sterile dressing and place it over the socket. Ask the victim to bite firmly on the pad for at least ten minutes to allow a clot to form.

Winding

Take action if any of the following occurs:

- Difficulty breathing
- Nausea
- Abdominal pain

What to look for:

- Inability to speak
- Obvious distress from abdominal pain
- Nausea or vomiting

A blow to the upper part of the abdomen can temporarily affect the solar plexus (a cluster of nerve fibres at the back of the abdominal cavity). Although painful and frightening, the effects of winding pass off quickly. But the victim may feel bruised for a few days.

1 As soon as the victim can move, help him or her into the most comfortable position possible. This is often sitting down or leaning on a table. Loosen clothing at chest and waist. Keep reassuring the person that the spasm will pass and breathing will become easier. DO NOT attempt to rub the abdomen or 'pump' the legs.

✚ **CALL AN AMBULANCE AS SOON AS POSSIBLE AND STAY WITH THE VICTIM UNTIL IT ARRIVES.**

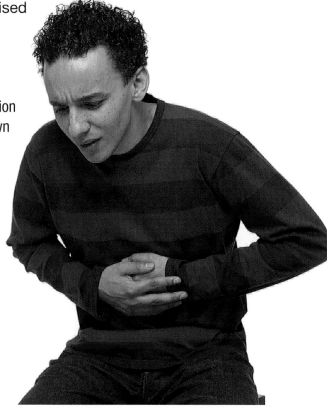

2 Do not give any food or drink to the victim until he or she is fully recovered, or has been assessed by a doctor in case of internal injuries.

✚ **ADVISE THE VICTIM TO SEEK MEDICAL ADVICE TO MAKE SURE THAT NO LASTING INTERNAL INJURY HAS OCCURRED.**

3 If the victim becomes unconscious, gently turn him or her onto the side and into the recovery position (see page 11). Clear and open the airway (see page 8). Give CPR (cardiopulmonary resuscitation, see page 13) if necessary.

Wrist injury

Injuries to the wrist occur frequently, especially after a fall onto an outstretched hand. Sprains of the wrist are common, and it can be hard to distinguish a sprain from a broken bone. A fracture of one of the tiny wrist bones, the scaphoid, may go undetected at first, leading to problems later on.

Take action if any of the following occurs:

- Obvious deformity of the wrist.
- Inability to move the hand normally.
- Fingertips turning blue.
- Inability to feel the ends of the fingers.

What to look for:

- Pain around the wrist
- Difficulty in moving the wrist or hand normally
- Swelling or bruising

1 Ask the victim to sit down and gently support the arm and wrist on the injured side. If necessary, treat any open wound (see page 34).

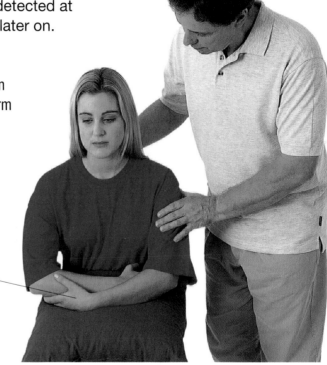

Rest the injured arm on a soft support such as a cushion.

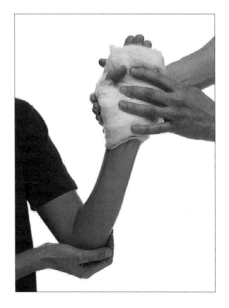

2 Arrange clean, soft padding around the injured area. Place a triangular bandage between the arm and the chest, and tie it up into a sling to support the arm (see page 28).

3 Keep the victim sitting down and arrange transport to hospital.

Index

Copyright © 2004
The Reader's Digest Association Limited,
11 Westferry Circus, Canary Wharf, London E14 4HE

Reader's Digest First Aid was first published as *First Aid* in the *Reader's Digest Complete A–Z of Medicine and Health* series by the Reader's Digest Association Ltd, London. It was commissioned, edited, designed and typeset for Reader's Digest Association by Librios Publishing, 21 Catherine Street, London WC2B 5JS
(email: bookcreation@librios.com)

FOR LIBRIOS PUBLISHING

PROJECT MANAGER	Finny Fox-Davies
DESIGN MANAGER	Justina Leitão
SENIOR DESIGNERS	Keith Miller; Rachel Riches; Beatriz Waller
EDITORIAL ASSISTANT	David Popey
EDITORS	Kim Davies; Cécile Landau
INDEXER	Marie Lorimer
PUBLISHING DIRECTOR	Hal Robinson
EDITORIAL DIRECTOR	Ali Moore
ART DIRECTOR	Peter Laws

FOR THE READER'S DIGEST

COMMISSIONING EDITOR	Jonathan Bastable
ART EDITORS	Louise Turpin; Joanna Walker
PRE-PRESS ACCOUNTS MANAGER	Penny Grose
EDITORIAL ASSISTANT	Lucy Murray

READER'S DIGEST GENERAL BOOKS

EDITORIAL DIRECTOR	Cortina Butler
MANAGING EDITOR	Alastair Holmes
ART DIRECTOR	Nick Clark
DEVELOPMENT EDITOR	Ruth Binney
SERIES EDITOR	Christine Noble

We are committed to both the quality of our products and the service we provide to our customers. We value your comments, so please feel free to contact us on 08705 113366 or via our website at:
www.readersdigest.co.uk

If you have any comments or suggestions about the content of our books, email us at **gbeditorial@readersdigest.co.uk**

Copyright ©2004 Reader's Digest Association Far East Limited
Philippines copyright ©2004 Reader's Digest Association Far East Limited

® Reader's Digest, The Digest and the Pegasus logo are registered trademarks of the Reader's Digest Association Inc., of Pleasantville, New York, USA.

Colour origination: Colour Systems, London
Printed and bound in Europe by Arvato Iberia

ISBN 0 276 42894 3
Book code 400-214-01

Picture credits:

New photography John Freeman

p. 38 (From top to bottom) Viewing Medicine, Wellcome Trust, Viewing Medicine, Wellcome Trust

Emergency numbers

Ambulance, Coastguard, Fire, Police	**999**
Doctor	
Surgery	
Out-of-hours	
Local Hospital	
NHS Direct	0845 4647
Dentist	
Surgery	
Out-of-hours	
Pharmacist	
Electricity	
Gas	
River authority	
Notes	

Calling for emergency help

If possible, stay with the casualty and ask a bystander to telephone for help. Give the following information:

- Your name and the telephone number you are calling from
- Location, as precisely as possible
- Type of incident
- The number, condition, approximate age and sex of casualties
- Any other risk factors

Observation notes

Note observations at ten minute intervals while waiting for medical help. Pass the notes to the doctor or paramedic, or send them with the casualty

Name

Date and Time

Eyes

This is a useful gauge for reaction while checking other responses

- Open spontaneously
- Open in response to voice
- Open in response to stimulus such as pinching
- No response

Speech

Speak clearly to the victim and listen carefully for a response

- Answers questions coherently
- Answers questions but confused
- Answers but words cannot be understood
- No response

Movement

Give verbal instructions for movement or apply physical stimulus such as pinching the skin

- Follows verbal instructions to move (a hand or foot)
- Can point to site of injury or pain
- Responds to physical stimulus
- No response

Pulse

Check: adult or child's pulse at wrist or neck; inner arm on a baby. Count the number of beats per minute and note the type

Strong	Weak
Regular	Irregular

Breathing

Count the number of breaths per minute and note the type

Quiet	Noisy
Easy	Difficult